AF682752

"A Whole Little City by Itself"

Tranquille and Tuberculosis

"A Whole Little City by Itself"

Tranquille and Tuberculosis

Wayne Norton

Plateau Press
Kamloops, British Columbia

Copyright @ Plateau Press 1999

Copyright Notice

All rights reserved. No part of this book may be reproduced in any form by any means without the prior written permission of the publisher, except by a reviewer, who may quote brief passages for review purposes.

Plateau Press
PO Box 283
Kamloops, British Columbia
V2C 5K6
Fax (250) 314-1803

Canadian Cataloguing in Publication Data

Norton, Wayne, 1948--
"A whole little city by itself"

Includes bibliographical references and index.
ISBN 0-9698842-4-9

1. King Edward Sanatorium (Tranquille, B.C.)--History.
2. British Columbia Anti-Tuberculosis Society--History.
3. Tuberculosis--British Columbia--History. I. Title.
RC309.5.C3N67 1999 362.1'96995'009711 C99-910686-4

Front cover photograph by Lake Denman (BCARS I-51951)

Printed in Canada by **Navigator Communications**

Plateau Press is distributed by: **Sandhill Book Marketing**
99-1270 Ellis Street
Kelowna, BC
V1Y 1Z4
Telephone (250) 763-1406
Fax (250) 763-4051

Contents

The Author

Wayne Norton was born in Calgary, and was educated in Canada and Scotland. He has written on the history of the prairie provinces, the Thompson River valley, East Kootenay and Scotland. A high school teacher in Kamloops, he is married with two adult children. *A Whole Little City by Itself* is his first venture into the history of health care in British Columbia.

Maps and Photographs

A map of the dry belt of British Columbia is found on page 29.

Photographs are found between pages 98 and 99 and between pages 156 and 157.

A map of the Tranquille site in the 1950s is found on page 170.

Dedication

The President and Directors of the British Columbia Lung Association take pride and pleasure in introducing *A Whole Little City by Itself: Tranquille and Tuberculosis*. The book is presented in recognition of the centennial of the Canadian Lung Association, which celebrates one hundred years of service to Canada in the year 2000.

This century has seen remarkable changes in medical theory and practice since the founding of the original Association for the Prevention of Consumption and Other Forms of Tuberculosis, from which the Canadian Lung Association has evolved. A provincial organization, the British Columbia Anti-Tuberculosis Society, was formed in 1904 and soon affiliated with the national body.

In commemorating the anniversary of the national organization, the British Columbia Lung Association welcomes the opportunity to draw attention to its own formative years. Recounted here is much of the history of the fight against tuberculosis in this province, during the first half of the century. The Association gratefully acknowledges the meticulous research and considerable effort of the author, and thanks him for allowing the predecessors of the British Columbia Lung Association to be acknowledged through his labours. This book is dedicated to their memory.

Marilyn Lawrence, President
British Columbia Lung Association

Foreword

The reader of this splendid story of the Tranquille Sanatorium near Kamloops, British Columbia will enjoy a well-written and carefully researched slice of provincial history with implications far beyond the immediate locale and its daily life. Opened in 1907, this was Canada's seventh sanatorium and the first west of Ontario. It was conceived in imitation of others spawned in Western Europe and North America at the turn of the century in the wake of a movement begun in Germany by Hermann Brehmer in 1854 at Gorbersdorf.

In this story lie many of the landmark steps taken by government in the creation of public health policy. As well, much in the behaviour of society in the early days of this century is laid bare. As the complex tale of personal motivations and political and regional interests emerges from the local community, from other people and parts of the province, from local, provincial and national governments and from the array of professionals, both medical and non-medical (architects, builders, engineers, agriculturists), one is brought face-to-face with the challenges of this endeavour and with the hard road of philanthropy and service, of bringing people and politicians to a common purpose, of personal sacrifice and selfless duty when there was not enough, as there seldom was. Over the busy scene of the providers hover the ghosts of patients past, with enduring memories of their hopes and fears, and their patient--at times, impatient--submission to the rather rigid discipline of the care. Present for all too many, was the inevitability of death, and sadly, the social stigma, the shame and isolation which tuberculosis carried and, regrettably, still carries. In *Below the Magic Mountain*, Linda Bryder aptly described their anguish. Tuberculosis, she comments, was "both the crime and the punishment."

All these facets of the founding of sanatoria, their maintenance and the life led by their patients were shared in some degree by all sanatoria, which widens the applicability of the story told here to the century-long movement. Norton's account is a reminder to the British Columbia Lung Association and to all non-governmental organizations that politics is not a world of facts but one of perceptions.

An important role of independent societies is the molding of these perceptions.

A Whole Little City by Itself projects a very human story and covers a broad canvas. In doing so, it reminds us of the limitations of a too-narrow reductionism in our concept of disease. The reality is that the expression and management of disease, especially tuberculosis, exists inescapably in the much wider context of society. Personal perceptions, money and politics, ambition and fashion, dogma, conviction and prejudice, hypocrisy and not least, procrastination and a poor appreciation of priority are all involved in the equation. In 1882, amidst all the excitement attending the discovery of the cause of tuberculosis, the Italian physician, Bacelli, cautioned, "The bacillus is not yet all there is to tuberculosis."

Hospitals devoted to the care and cure of tuberculosis have a long and well-intentioned history. But the antimicrobial era put an end to their usefulness and was inexpressibly good news for those who suffered from this disease. Almost overnight a commonly fatal disease became fatal only rarely, curable in almost all cases within months with no need for hospitalization for the great majority.

If compassion and caring were the only good they did, this would have amply justified the efforts of those who created the "sans." It is fitting that we pay them tribute, important that we learn from their experience, and important that we not forget.

Edward A. Allen, MB, Ch.B., F.R.C.P.(C), F.C.C.P.
Former Director, Tuberculosis Control,
Ministry of Health, British Columbia

Author's Preface and Acknowledgements

I was a resident of Kamloops for twenty years before I became curious about the Tranquille site. The buildings were still in use by the Department of Mental Health when I arrived here, and I suppose my assumption was that the history of the old sanatorium was known to others, if not to me. As my research began, I found the accepted history of the institution to be an amalgam of myth, misunderstanding and conflicting fact. At the conclusion of this process, I am hopeful that I have separated successfully at least some of the strands of fact and fiction . However, I am also struck by how quickly historical knowledge can erode and disintegrate. The records of the Tranquille Sanatorium and the Anti-Tuberculosis Society remain accessible, it is true, but they can now only occasionally be supplemented by the knowledge of people who worked at the institution until 1958. With memory and experience still fresh, a more complete history could have been created during the decade after the closure of Tranquille. More than forty years later, the reconstruction of that history—especially of the human aspects of the story—has sometimes seemed out of reach. It is as if the historical knowledge of the institution has become comparable to the remaining buildings at Tranquille: closed up, in disrepair, and on the verge of disappearing completely. It is my hope that these pages have managed to rescue a portion of that history.

I have incurred many debts of gratitude over the three years this study has occupied. Many people, simply with a question or a suggestion along the way, made me aware of unexplored possibilities and unanticipated perspectives. Others assisted by relating personal experiences, searching for photographs, and explaining the operation of an institution in terms understandable to one with no medical knowledge and no personal experience of Tranquille. I have been fortunate enough to speak to people who were children at Tranquille in the 1920s, and to people who worked there in the 1940s and 1950s. Everyone stated that Tranquille was a place unlike any other—a good place to grow up, an institution with a unique working atmosphere, even a remarkable place to be a patient.

I must acknowledge the assistance of many people. The staff at the Kamloops Museum and Archives managed to maintain their cheerful expressions through what must have seemed an endless series of requests for assistance. Scott McDonald at the British Columbia Lung Association was consistently helpful, even when the timing of my visits was less than convenient. John Stewart and David Mattison are two of the many archivists who provided assistance at the British Columbia Archives and Records Service. Bill Rawling at National Defence Headquarters in Ottawa, Wendy Hunt at the British Columbia Medical Association Archives, and Lee Perry at the Charles Woodward Memorial Room at the University of British Columbia all took time to assist.

I want particularly to thank Joan Best and Barb Derenowsky for their sustained interest and moral support. Terry Munson had the patience to listen to endless speculation about sundry points of research as we enjoyed walking at Tranquille. For assistance, information or photographs, I am grateful to Glennis Zilm, Ethel Warbinek, Alice De Marni, Naomi Miller, Brian Ross, Mike Scramstad, Dave and Jan Davies, Tony and Paula Walters, Alex McIntosh, Verna Vanclieaf, Fred and Rowna Weys, Madelaine Webber, Joan Newman, Dana and Jade Norton, Bill Henderson, Andrew Yarmie, Ethel Busch, Marianne Trestain, Kash Dhaliwal, Jan Antons, Peter Walters, Skip Seymour, Kelly Nolin, Dr. David Stewart, and Dr. Ted Allen. Personal interviews were particularly valuable in providing information that is not found in the public record. For granting those interviews, I thank Joan Best, Marlene Freeman, Bette Wood, Dr. William McLaren, Gerry Rositch, Les and Margaret King, Ray and Ivy Quinville, and Eva Moody. Patricia Koretchuk was kind enough to allow me to read the chapter about Tranquille in the biography of David Caldow she is preparing. Jeanne M. Des Mazes provided insight into patient life at the sanatorium. Nikolas Cuff and Wilf Schmidt donated much time and skill in working with the photographs. However, none of this assistance would have been enough without the encouragement of my wife Val, whose support I particularly and gratefully acknowledge.

Financial assistance contributed significantly to the process of creating this book. A research trip to the National Archives of Canada was made possible by a travel grant from the J.S. Ewart Memorial Fund administered by the University of Manitoba. A grant from the British Columbia Lung Association substantially assisted with publication and printing expenses. The board of directors of the Kamloops Museum Association provided a level of encouragement that was equally as important as the welcome financial contributions. If, despite all this assistance, the present volume does not convey a sense of the unique experience of Tranquille, the fault cannot be attributed to those who favoured me with their assistance and reminiscences. Nor can any difficulties with historical accuracy be attributed to them. For any errors or omissions, I alone must bear responsibility.

The present study is offered not as a look at what could be, but rather as a look at what once was. In British Columbia, elements of the medical and philanthropic communities of a young and dynamic province combined to create a remarkable society and a remarkable institution. Modern charitable organizations in British Columbia owe a debt to the British Columbia Anti-Tuberculosis Society that, for too long, has been unacknowledged. The institution established by the society—the Tranquille Sanatorium near Kamloops—stands today under threat of demolition. Few remember that, under private and government administration, the institution provided fifty years of care to victims of tuberculosis. Few understand that the sanatorium represented the local chapter in a story of national and international dimensions.

The disease the society and the sanatorium were created to combat can no longer be ignored. The history of the British Columbia Anti-Tuberculosis Society and the sanatorium at Tranquille reveals much about the social, political and medical past of British Columbia. That story, too, should no longer be ignored.

Wayne Norton
Kamloops, British Columbia
June 1999

The Captain of all These Men of Death

Future historians may well conclude that the defining attribute of the twentieth century has been its belief in progress and improvement. Though the belief has suffered setbacks, it manages to rebound with each generation and at the end of the century holds the same pre-eminence it held at the beginning. The citizens of the modern Western world believe that the lessons of the past have been learned. We hold that the human race is intelligent enough not to repeat those mistakes, and that there will be no need to confront tomorrow problems that were vanquished yesterday. Conveniently ignored is the fact that humankind is not always in control of events. We forget that situations have ways of repeating themselves in different guises. We try to forget that the twentieth century provides plenty of evidence that humanity does not readily learn from past experience.

Improvements in medical science have contributed significantly to this belief in steady progress. Whether in rich nations or poor, people live longer lives due to the ability of medicine to identify and often cure what ails them. Victory has been declared in battles against diseases that once claimed a heavy toll of human life. Because of medical knowledge and treatments, measles, diphtheria, leprosy, and smallpox are afflictions that no longer hold the element of terror they once possessed. However, evidence is emerging to suggest that at least some of our advances and triumphs may prove to be of temporary duration. Most frightening is the current dramatic resurgence of a disease that has defied humanity for thousands of years. The disease was the chief cause of death century after century, yet it is now oddly absent from the collective memory of Western nations. While a lesser disease like polio is well remembered and well documented, tuberculosis is the forgotten killer.

The genus Mycobacterium, to which the species causing tuberculosis belongs, may have existed since the origins of life itself. Other bacteria have been found to exist in rocks estimated to be three thousand million years old, while the first evidence of bacterial infection dates from about 40,000 years ago. There are indications that tuberculosis exacted its toll of human life during the Stone Age and that the ancient Egyptians suffered from the disease. Different societies gave the disease different names, but always the idea of wasting away was at the heart of the terminology. Consumption and phthisis were terms used from biblical and Hippocratic times. In the nineteenth century, the term tuberculosis was adopted by the medical profession, and the name White Plague also came into use after Oliver Wendell Holmes, Sr. coined the term in 1861. Though the Black Death had a more profound effect over a shorter period, tuberculosis took such a steady toll of human life that it might be regarded as humanity's greatest killer. In the cities of Europe, during each of the three centuries before our own, the disease was the cause of as many as one death out of five. Tuberculosis is suspected to have existed in parts of Africa and Asia for thousands of years, and in the Americas well before the arrival of the Europeans.

There has always been a sense of mystery about tuberculosis and its cause has been subject to varied interpretations. This was partly due to the variety of its manifestations. Though pulmonary tuberculosis is its most prevalent form, the disease also commonly attacks the throat, the bowels, ovaries, and bones. In fact, teeth are the only part of the body spared. As its cause was unknown, curious attitudes and attributions developed, particularly in the nineteenth century. Mothers' milk, for example, was regarded for a time as a particularly effective treatment.

While the disease had been previously romanticized to some extent, people in the early nineteenth century went further and elevated sufferers to a higher plane of existence. Many people believed that to suffer from tuberculosis conferred on the victim sensitivity and distinction unattainable by those blessed with good health. So numerous were the writers and artists who contracted the disease (though it was no more prevalent amongst them than amongst the general population), the view developed that somehow their suffering was the wellspring of the great art they produced. Even those not afflicted often adopted the languor associated with tuberculosis as a proof they possessed artistic talents. To die young of tuberculosis was to be on the side of the angels. The list of victims reads like a catalogue of famous names from nineteenth century art, literature, music, and politics. Amongst dozens of others, the list includes Keats, Chopin, the Bronte sisters, Dostoevsky, and Gaugin. For those who held this view, the fact that a disproportionate number of the poor suffered from the disease was proof only that a form of gentility was available through channels other than birth alone.

Others held the contrary view that to suffer from tuberculosis was to reveal a weakness of character or of heredity. Therefore, those who suffered from the disease were either themselves to blame for their situation or beyond help. This enabled many in the middle and upper classes to insist that the poor should help themselves, and reduced their enthusiasm for the medical crusade against tuberculosis. The poor achieved no fame through their suffering and undoubtedly would have disdained a philosophy that admired them for their illness. With feelings of guilt added to the suffering the disease entailed, they could only wonder at a theory that blamed them for having been selected as the victims.

Until the late nineteenth century, there was much speculation about the nature and cause of the disease. Generally regarded as a "wet" disease, tuberculosis was associated with damp, urban life and moist climates. Overcrowding and enclosed spaces were identified as contributing factors. Florence Nightingale, for example, believed tuberculosis was "induced by the foul air of houses." Quite logically, therefore, the treatment of tuberculosis came to include the avoidance of foul air, damp weather, and cities. Doctors advised those patients whose financial circumstances would allow it to seek dry air on islands and deserts, to travel to mountains and southern climates, or to seek the clean, crisp cold of a Canadian winter. It was from this outlook that the sanatorium movement emerged. In Germany and Switzerland , isolated treatment centres initially were located at high altitudes away from urban centres, where victims of tuberculosis could be protected from everyday stress and from the demands of family and career. In such remote and cheerful surroundings, a healthy diet, fresh air, and rest could combine to provide the best chance of recovery. Though offering no guarantees, the sanatorium did offer at least some hope to people who knew that to contract tuberculosis was usually to receive a death sentence.

In 1882, Robert Koch stunned the medical world with his discovery of the tubercle bacillus. He demonstrated that the century's deadliest disease was caused by a bacterial infection. The discovery destroyed or undermined all previous theories of tuberculosis, but it also gave further impetus to the sanatorium movement. If the disease was indeed communicable as demonstrated by Koch, then society's best interests lay in isolating those who suffered from it. If early intervention could save lives, it was important to offer a full treatment to those in early stages of the disease. The antituberculosis movement became another example of late Victorian and Edwardian philanthropy, in Britain and throughout the Empire. As such, it carried with it the accompanying air of a crusade against an enemy that could be beaten. By the end of the nineteenth century, Canadian doctors, too, were adopting the European faith that the sanatorium system was the most effective way to combat tuberculosis.

It is not surprising that the major population centres of the province saw the emergence of the movement in British Columbia. Victoria, in particular, took the lead in initiating British Columbia's antituberculous campaign. The stubborn belief in the healing properties of dry air, the route of the Canadian Pacific Railway, and the wish to locate sanatoria away from population centres were all factors in the process. Almost inevitably, the dry belt from Lytton to Kamloops became the area of choice. Kamloops and Tranquille, Victoria and later Vancouver would be the centres around which the local variation of a national and international story developed. In British Columbia, like elsewhere, the tale includes its share of hope and triumph. But disappointment and bitterness, suspicion and malice play parts that are disturbingly significant. It is a story that includes elements of public fear, private shame, government action, and government inaction. It is a story that has striking parallels with the attitudes and controversies surrounding AIDS as the century ends.

The twentieth century has seen notable figures felled by tuberculosis, but, with the exceptions of George Orwell, Eleanor Roosevelt and actress Vivien Leigh, they are primarily figures from the pre-World War II years. Thomas Mann writes of the disease in *The Magic Mountain*, while Franz Kafka and Katherine Mansfield have also added their literary comments. Jazz musician Charlie Christian and country singer Jimmy Rodgers were both claimed by tuberculosis. Rodgers would have been the worst nightmare of a sanatorium. He chain-smoked, drank heavily, and refused to compromise with his illness, dying of tuberculosis at a young age.

In the latter half of this century, the human experience with tuberculosis has been forgotten. Until now, the greater attention recently given to AIDS and to a variety of so-called super-germs has not allowed the significance of the recurrence of tuberculosis to sink into the public consciousness. Yet, the World Health Organization and other observers believe that the greatest scourge known to humanity is on the verge of reclaiming its historic pre-eminence.

It seems unlikely these predictions are mistaken, at least in the developing world. If the predictions prove to be correct, however, it is unlikely that sanatoria will witness a revival. They were the front line of defence against tuberculosis and quite possibly played a significant role in the slow but steady reduction in death rates during the first half of the this century. Nevertheless, it has been difficult to assess their exact contribution to the decline in mortality rates before the advent of the antimicrobial drugs. By isolating sufferers, they protected society and permitted some victims at least to survive the disease. Though hospices are being created today for AIDS victims, these facilities are located in urban centres. Society is unlikely to accept again the notion that tuberculosis sufferers should be exiled to distant locations. The belief in the healing powers of dry climates and higher elevations is now regarded as a discredited myth of a bygone era. Despite the current concern with super-bugs, the public's faith in the ability of medical science to provide effective drug treatments is undiminished. Unfortunately, so is the public's reluctance to provide adequate funding. Nevertheless, it is to medical scientific research, not sanatoria, that society will look to combat resurgent tuberculosis.

The optimism prevalent at the beginning of this century contrasts with the discouragement of many working in the medical field today. Perhaps the experience of the people discussed in these pages will hold some lessons for us as we combat the scourges of our day and as we turn to face an old enemy once more. Tuberculosis has shown itself a very clever bacterium—able to transform itself quickly to outmanoeuvre the drugs that human science has developed to kill it. Tuberculosis has emerged once again as a dangerous predator, capable of resisting the antimicrobial drugs that just a few years ago came so close to eradicating the disease altogether from industrialized countries. AIDS and tuberculosis are linked, and it is not a coincidence that concurrent epidemics are sweeping the world, especially in Asia and sub-Saharan Africa. With the emergence of AIDS in European countries and North America, the tuberculosis rate has been rising steadily since the early 1980s. Recent reports suggest the former Soviet Union will experience particular difficulties. Tuberculosis does not respect international boundaries.

Widespread misuse of prescribed drugs, increased immigration, international travel, and general ignorance of the history of tuberculosis have combined to allow the tubercle bacilli to return in strength. A century ago, that strength was universally acknowledged. However, many in the medical community began to insist that it could not remain unchallenged.

Philanthropy and Provincialism

In every Canadian province at the dawn of the century, a handful of medical practitioners and their supporters believed that a campaign against tuberculosis should be undertaken immediately. They argued that the White Plague could be defeated, and that it was the duty of private citizens and governments to rise to the challenge by employing modern medical knowledge and techniques. Encouraged by expressions of support for their goals, the crusaders optimistically turned to the mundane details of public education and fund-raising, and to the more contentious problem of selecting sanatorium construction sites. Everywhere they were to find their optimism and enthusiasm sorely tested.

Central to the antituberculous campaign of the early century was the proposal that sanatoria for the treatment of incipient cases should be established throughout Canada. Like most beliefs held by early Canadian antituberculous campaigners, this approach was derived largely from European research and experience, particularly that of Germany and Switzerland. The first German sanatorium was opened in the 1854 and others followed. They attracted the attention of doctors in other European countries, and they were widely imitated. However, it was only when American doctor Edward L. Trudeau established North America's first modern sanatorium near Lake Saranac in the Adirondack Mountains in 1885 that the European influence spread to this continent.

The Sanatorium Movement in Canada

In Canada, the movement had its first successes in Ontario. As early as 1889, an Anti-Consumption League was formed in Toronto. In 1896, a group of Toronto activists formed the ambitiously named National Sanitarium Association, with the financial support of publisher William Gage and industrial magnate Hart Massey.

Following the lead of their European and American counterparts, the association believed that tuberculosis could best be treated by isolating its victims in environments where proper care would be provided by trained medical staff. The association announced its intention to build Canada's first sanatorium. It considered a number of sites, including Kamloops in British Columbia, and Medicine Hat and Moose Jaw in what was then the North West Territories. However, when the town of Gravenhurst in the Muskoka region north of Toronto offered a financial inducement of $10,000, the association decided to build Canada's first sanatorium there. The Muskoka Cottage Sanitarium for fee-paying patients was opened in the summer of 1897.[1]

Despite its name, the National Sanitarium Association was essentially an Ontario-based organization, with some involvement by Montreal's anglophone medical community. Though its board of governors would have preferred the institution to be of a national character, nearly all patients were from Ontario. Of 147 patients being treated in 1899, 136 were from Ontario, nine were from other Canadian provinces, and two were from the United States. In its advertising, the association made much of the fact that tuberculosis was "especially a disease of the poor," but admission to the Muskoka Cottage Sanitarium was denied those unable to pay the fees.[2]

Though the beginning made by the National Sanitarium Association was applauded, many thought treatment should be more readily available to sufferers in other provinces and to the poor. A committee was appointed by the Canadian Medical Association (CMA) in 1899 to consider methods of combatting tuberculosis, and, at its annual meeting in September 1900, the CMA formed the Association for the Prevention of Tuberculosis. Encouraged to broaden the association by Governor General the Earl of Minto, the CMA sponsored a conference in Ottawa on 14 February 1901. Though most of those in attendance came from Ontario and Quebec, there was a healthy representation from the rest of Canada. Wanting to cover all eventualities, the new organization named itself, in rather cumbersome fashion, the Canadian Association for the Prevention of Consumption and Other Forms of Tuberculosis.

By establishing an organization that was national in more than name only, the new association sought to educate the public about the nature of the disease and about the best methods of combatting it. Because of its successful publicity campaign, considerable discussion concerning tuberculosis appeared in newspapers from coast to coast. In 1902, a second sanatorium, the Muskoka Free Hospital for Consumptives, was opened by the National Sanitarium Association in Gravenhurst for non-paying patients. By 1903, a handful of Canadian cities had passed by-laws prohibiting spitting in public places. Discussion of the merits of sanatorium treatment continued to hold the public's attention, as the association sought to persuade the federal government that it had a role to play in fighting a disease that did not recognize provincial boundaries.

However, in drawing the disease to the attention of the public, the influence of the new association should not be over estimated. Tuberculosis was already regarded with universal horror. It was widely acknowledged as the most prevalent cause of death in both Europe and North America throughout the nineteenth century. On that score, the public needed little education. "Cures" for consumption were advertised in newspapers as broadly as elixirs for grippe and hair restoration. Doctor Barnham's Pink Pills for Pale People was just one of the more amusingly-named remedies offered to victims who knew that the disease was no laughing matter, that one in nine deaths in Canada was attributable to tuberculosis, and that no cure yet existed.

It was widely believed, however, that the disease could be treated successfully in its early stages and that the right climate could make a world of difference. In the late nineteenth century, the American states of Arizona, New Mexico and California were thought to possess dry climates particularly suited to improving the condition of consumptives. Many a pale Briton (especially those in possession of a little wealth) appeared in the American southwest hoping to benefit from the invigorating climate, and often hoping to indulge in a little bit of cowboy life at the same time.

Kamloops Steps Forward

In 1895, the question of the location of a national sanatorium was being examined by those who would soon found the National Sanitarium Association. The drier sections of the Canadian prairies and the British Columbia interior were scrutinized for their ability to provide a beneficial climate for the treatment of tuberculosis. In typical western Canadian fashion, the local board of trade and the region's newspaper at each prospective sanatorium location combined to insist that their community alone possessed all the attributes necessary for the establishment of a successful institution.

With the virtues of Regina, Moose Jaw, and Medicine Hat being touted by their respective local boosters, the recently incorporated city of Kamloops took the opportunity to express its own civic pride. A committee of citizens and local doctors produced a pamphlet calculated to influence the National Sanitarium Association in its site selection process. The pamphlet presented Kamloops' "pre-eminent claim" to treat tuberculosis more beneficially than any place north of the Mexican border. With its air and water of "unusual purity," Kamloops was said to be "better than Egypt" and destined to be home to the "Sanitorium of the North."[3] John Davie, one of five doctors appointed to British Columbia's inaugural Board of Health late in 1895, declared in his first official speech as a board member that a sanatorium should be built near Kamloops.[4]

The Kamloops *Inland Sentinel* agreed, expressing the opinion that few places possessed "greater advantages" for the treatment of tuberculosis than Kamloops.[5] Visitors from eastern Canada interested in the emerging antituberculous movement agreed. Peter Bryce, secretary of the Ontario Provincial Board of Health, visited the Thompson region as part of a North American tour to investigate potential sanatorium sites. He stated that Kamloops was the best location in Canada, if not in the whole of North America. In February 1896, he formally recommended Kamloops to British Columbia's medical officials as the ideal site for a sanatorium, stating that he was "charmed by Kamloops as a health resort for consumptives."[6]

With the selection of Gravenhurst in 1896 as the site of the first sanatorium, nothing came of the recommendation at the time, but the Kamloops region continued to interest sanatorium proponents.

While visiting the area in May 1899, Montreal-area M.P. Dr. Thomas Roddick, accompanied by CPR president William Van Horne, made a special trip to Tranquille, thirteen kilometres west of Kamloops on the north shore of the lake. At Tranquille, they visited two pioneers who occasionally supplemented their ranch incomes by providing room and board for victims of tuberculosis. Roddick was reported to say on his return that there was "no more suitable spot in North America for a sanatorium than in the vicinity of Tranquille."[7]

In Kamloops itself, the antituberculosis crusade found a local champion in Dr. Arthur Procter, the young medical officer of the Royal Inland Hospital. Described as a "progressive member of his profession," Procter combined his private practice with official duties for the Royal Inland Hospital, the CPR, the Provincial Home for Old Men, and the Provincial Jail.[8] With interest in the possibilities presented by a Kamloops-area sanatorium sustained by reports of the move to form a new national antituberculosis society, Procter suggested the Inland Board of Trade should appoint a committee to investigate the question.

The committee reported enthusiastically in late January 1901. Doctor Procter provided statistics to show that the city was beneficial for consumptive patients. He stated that, of the forty-four cases of pulmonary tuberculosis he had treated during his three years of local practice, twenty-nine were either cured or much improved. He noted that the fifteen people who had died all arrived in poor condition and "would have died anyway."[9] Another local doctor provided further statistics to show how well consumptives responded to the local climate, speculating that perhaps at Kamloops "the hot dry days of summer with their bright sunlight kill the bacilli and sterilize the dust of the town."

Despite the muted reservations of some members, the Inland Board of Trade approved the committee's recommendation that a sanatorium should be established locally. The decision was particularly significant, as the Board of Trade was largely synonymous with the city government. The city's political and business communities, therefore, were in support of the proposal. Decisions were made to lobby both the provincial and federal governments to support the establishment of a sanatorium in

Kamloops and to seek the endorsement of the Associated Boards of Trade of British Columbia. Dr. Procter did not hesitate to draw the attention of his colleagues to the need for action on pulmonary tuberculosis when he attended the first meeting of the British Columbia Medical Association in Vancouver in 1901.[10] Procter also hoped to attend the first annual meeting of the Canadian Medical Association's new antituberculosis organization in Ottawa as the representative of a city united behind the idea of having a sanatorium located at Kamloops.

However, local opposition to the proposal surfaced immediately. Fearing a decision to locate a sanatorium at Kamloops would be made at the Ottawa conference, Kamloops doctor M.S. Wade wrote to the organizers. He stated most emphatically that the Inland Board of Trade resolution had been hastily arrived at by relying too heavily on the opinions of "book learned men in the East," a clear reference to Peter Bryce and Thomas Roddick. He argued that, because the proposed sanatorium would soon be filled to capacity, hundreds of tubercular individuals attracted to the region by the sanatorium would be forced to live amongst the healthy population of Kamloops. Consequently, he claimed, local workers would be infected and pushed from employment by "a horde of disease stricken unfortunates," and the business and real estate interests of the town would suffer dramatically. Wade insisted that a sanatorium should not be located in any town anywhere, and asked that delegates at the conference be made aware that the dry belt of British Columbia was far wider than just Kamloops.[11]

Though the *Inland Sentinel* remained supportive of the Board of Trade's position, the new *Kamloops Standard* newspaper warned that the community would be well-advised to acquaint itself with the drawbacks, arguing that the city should not let its "judgement be warped by the pathetic appeals of the parsons and fearful pictures of woe of the doctors."[12] Like M.S. Wade, the *Standard* painted a picture of contagion and civic decline, suggesting that the supposed benefits were much over-stated:

> It is hard to see how a sanatorium would benefit anybody but the inmates. If Kamloops is wishing to advertise itself for its philanthropy, it is doing a most

> Christian act, but most of the people here have come to chase the elusive dollar and can hardly yet afford to be philanthropic.[13]

With evident approval, the newspaper reported that the *Nelson Tribune* had "too much regard for Kamloops to be instrumental in making it the battleground for any contest with the white death," and therefore had refused to print an article submitted by the Inland Board of Trade favouring the establishment of a sanatorium in Kamloops. With approval even more evident, its editorial columns applauded California's proposed legislation to deny consumptives entry into the state. When Procter asked city council to send a Board of Trade delegation to Ottawa to urge the antituberculosis conference to locate a sanatorium at Kamloops—a request which seemed assured of success just three weeks earlier—he was turned down abruptly. One council member stated bluntly that he would approve of city money being spent only if the delegation were to lobby for a sanatorium to be built anywhere other than in Kamloops.[14]

Reports from the organizational meeting of the Canadian Association for the Prevention of Consumption and Other Forms of Tuberculosis in Ottawa suggested that climate was not necessarily the significant factor it was once believed to be. The news gave further encouragement to those opposed to locating a sanatorium in Kamloops. There followed a confusing month of lobbying, allegation, counter-allegation, approval by the Associated Boards of Trade of the original Kamloops position and demands for its withdrawal. To end the confusion, the city and the Inland Board of Trade agreed that it was necessary to send a delegation to Victoria. However, its mandate was to be radically different from that originally contemplated. The delegates were directed to press for changes to the *Health Act* to combat more effectively the spread of tuberculosis. They were also instructed to state clearly that Kamloops was not lobbying for the establishment of a sanatorium in its vicinity.

If delegates C.S. Stevens, Marsh Gordon, and Arthur Procter arrived in Victoria in mid-March somewhat uncertain of the direction their representations were to take, their discomfort is understandable. All were supporters of the original proposal to seek the establishment of a sanatorium in Kamloops, but after the turmoil of the last month, they may have believed themselves to be the only three local residents still favouring that position. They were in Victoria to advocate a course of inaction, certainly an unusual situation for any delegation on any topic.

In the provincial capital, Procter knew that, in some influential circles at least, his personal representations would be favourably received. Doctor Charles Fagan, British Columbia's first permanent Medical Health Officer, had not yet been in the job for two years. He was known to be a man of considerable energy, increasingly interested in the growing crusade against the White Plague. He had just returned from the initial meeting of the Canadian Association for the Prevention of Consumption and Other Forms of Tuberculosis in Ottawa, where he had taken an active role. He had addressed the convention on the need for women to abandon the fashion of long dresses, as such garments spread and collected all manner of infection by sweeping the "foul sidewalks" of Canadian cities. He spoke with approval of Victoria-area cleaners who refused to accept long dresses for laundering. The convention was impressed, and Fagan returned to Victoria as one of the new organization's table officers.

Doctor Fagan was keenly interested in the idea of establishing a sanatorium in the dry belt of British Columbia, most specifically in the vicinity of the Canadian Pacific line between Kamloops and Lytton. News that the board of trade of a dry-belt community was on record favouring the establishment of such an institution locally would have been welcome news indeed. However, both Fagan and Procter were deeply concerned by the ongoing newspaper agitation and the growing opposition to the idea from Kamloops. Not content simply to editorialize, the editor of the *Kamloops Standard* privately circulated a petition opposing the location of a sanatorium in Kamloops. With the signatures of forty Kamloops businessmen, four aldermen and three former mayors, it was published and sent to the Provincial Board of Health while the Kamloops delegation was still in Victoria.[15] Reports in the Victoria newspapers that the Kamloops delegation was advocating the location of a sanatorium in Kamloops resulted in the publication of another broadside by the *Standard*. When the chastened delegates returned from Victoria, they insisted that they had lobbied only for changes to the *Health Act* as directed and for the location of a sanatorium somewhere in the dry belt—not in Kamloops specifically. Fagan and Procter were learning quickly that the location of a sanatorium would be a controversial matter indeed.

The Kamloops delegation could at least claim some success for its lobbying efforts in Victoria. Policies suggested by the delegation were adopted by the provincial government in regulations proclaimed on 14 November 1901. Tuberculosis was made a reportable disease, while spitting in public buildings and tramways became a summary offence. Though often content to follow the example of Ontario, the province of British Columbia anticipated Ontario making tuberculosis a reportable disease by more than a decade.[16] The new regulations represented, more than anything, the growing influence of Doctor Fagan. With the government moving in the right direction, Fagan began to urge it to embrace the principle that government should build and operate a sanatorium as part of its responsibility for public health. Predictably, the *Kamloops Standard* had something to say on the matter:

> No Government has yet accepted the socialistic idea that the poor should be doctored gratis, though it is a good one, and they will hate to create a precedent that will mean a largely increased expenditure.[17]

Nevertheless, the view was widely shared that the government was on the verge of making an announcement.

Such speculation was given further credence in June 1902, when the Victoria newspapers reported that the federal and provincial governments and the CPR had agreed to share the costs of construction of a tuberculosis sanatorium at Kamloops. Though incorrect, the announcement was a clear indication that Kamloops was still considered the most likely location for a sanatorium. Fagan was so encouraged by private assurances from members of the provincial government that he advised the attorney general, in his annual report for 1902, that an ideal site, protected from dust and north winds, had been selected at Kamloops some two to three miles up the North Thompson River.[18] He went further. In September 1903, he confided to the secretary of the Canadian Association for the Prevention of Consumption and Other Forms of Tuberculosis that construction of a sanatorium at Kamloops was likely to begin in the spring.[19]

Aware of these plans at least in part, many local residents continued to re-examine their initial enthusiasm of 1895. Before long, the previously supportive *Inland Sentinel* joined the ranks of those opposed to a local sanatorium. In an editorial generally critical of "high-salaried" civil servants, the *Sentinel* took the opportunity to declare specifically that the $3,600 paid to the provincial health officer was "a stipend out of all proportion to the work done" by Dr. Fagan.[20] This unusual attack proved to be the opening volley in a renewed campaign against the location of a sanatorium at Kamloops. Both local newspapers reflected the increasingly strong local opposition to the position taken by the Inland Board of Trade two years earlier.

The provincial government continued to avoid a clear and public commitment to the construction of a sanatorium. Perhaps recognizing that a public campaign would be necessary after all, those committed to the cause of fighting tuberculosis organized a large public meeting at the municipal building in Victoria on 20 January 1904. In attendance were the mayors of Vancouver, Victoria and Nanaimo, Premier Richard McBride, ministers of various denominations and several medical figures. Dr. Fagan addressed the gathering, noting that "man's most destructive enemy" claimed two hundred lives in British Columbia every year. He said that the federal government spent a great deal of money to combat bovine tuberculosis in the interests of Canada's agricultural reputation, but not a penny to alleviate human suffering from tuberculosis. Fagan then formally introduced a motion to found an organization to combat tuberculosis in British Columbia. Premier McBride quickly rose to second the motion and noted that Kamloops seemed to be a good site for a sanatorium. Also present was Dr. Procter, who agreed that consumptives were attracted to Kamloops, but added that there were no facilities available for treatment there. The meeting overwhelmingly endorsed the proposal to form a provincial organization, set membership fees at $1 per year, and formed a committee to lobby federal and provincial governments for building funds. An executive was elected headed by Procter as president and Fagan as secretary.

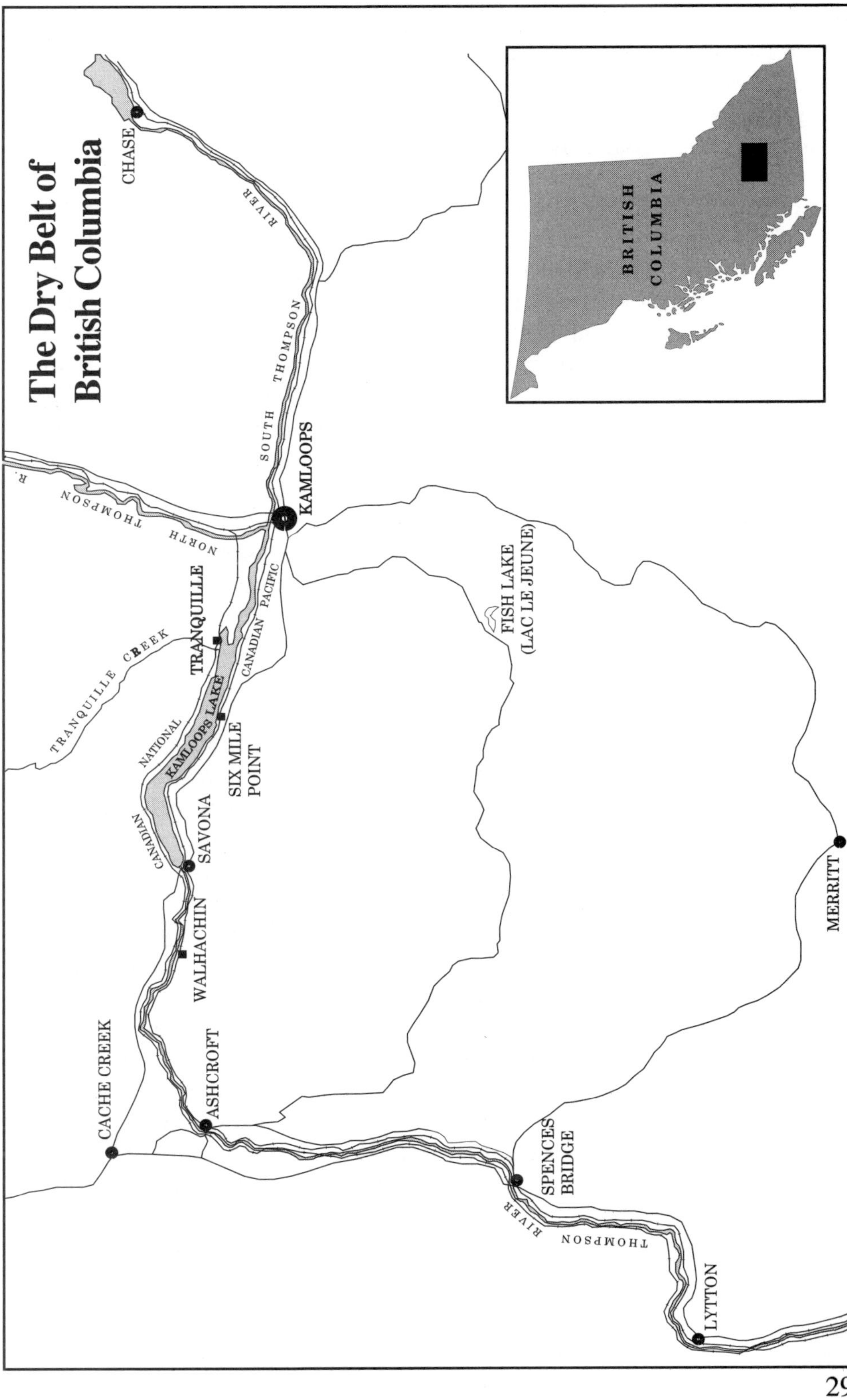
The Dry Belt of British Columbia
CHASE
RIVER
SOUTH THOMPSON
KAMLOOPS
NORTH THOMPSON R.
TRANQUILLE
TRANQUILLE CREEK
CANADIAN PACIFIC
KAMLOOPS LAKE
NATIONAL
CANADIAN
SIX MILE POINT
SAVONA
WALHACHIN
ASHCROFT
CACHE CREEK
FISH LAKE (LAC LE JEUNE)
MERRITT
SPENCES BRIDGE
RIVER
THOMPSON
LYTTON
BRITISH COLUMBIA

With its primary aim the establishment of a provincial tuberculosis sanatorium, the British Columbia Anti-Tuberculosis Society would waste no time in setting about its work. Seeing an opportunity, the president of the Ashcroft Power and Light Company also lost no time in making the new association an attractive offer. Soon after the founding meeting in Victoria, John Shields announced that his company would donate ten acres for a sanatorium at Boston Flats near Ashcroft. He added that it would also provide free water and light for a period of five years. Shield's proposal received further attention several weeks later when Fagan returned from Ottawa, where he had attended the third annual meeting of the Canadian Association for the Prevention of Consumption. Fagan reported that a delegation had met with Prime Minister Laurier, who promised federal assistance if investigation by the minister of justice found such a donation to be constitutional. The delegation also met with CPR president Sir Thomas Shaughnessy, who (rather more concretely) had donated $5,000 towards the establishment of a sanatorium in British Columbia.[21] To pressure the provincial government and to publicize its work, the provincial society erected tents behind the legislature in Victoria to treat patients during the summer.

Clearly, events were moving rapidly, and sanatorium opponents in Kamloops were alarmed. The Inland Board of Trade formally withdrew its earlier support for locating a sanatorium at Kamloops, and at its quarterly meeting in August threw its entire influence against such an eventuality. Nearly every businessman in Kamloops signed a petition pledging to support the fledgling British Columbia Anti-Tuberculosis Society "both morally and financially, as far as possible," but objecting to the location of a sanatorium within twenty-five miles of the city. M.S. Wade, by this time a member of the Board of Trade, stated that plans to send Fagan's tuberculosis tents to Kamloops would simply encourage consumptives to move to Kamloops. Another member, alderman George Loney warned the city was about to become "a Lazar house of consumptives," and a special committee was struck to present to civic, provincial and federal governments the views of the hastily-formed but aptly-named Anti-Sanitarium (in Kamloops) League.[22] Vancouver newspapers reported that ninety-five percent of Kamloops' business community supported the new league, and that individuals amongst them had promised to burn the tents should they be sent to Kamloops.[23]

Both Kamloops newspapers supported the new league. The *Standard*, echoing the revised Board of Trade position, urged residents of Kamloops to subscribe to the British Columbia Anti-Tuberculosis Society, but only if the sanatorium was located elsewhere, and warned that a sanatorium would attract hundreds of consumptives to Kamloops—far more than the proposed sanatorium could accommodate. The *Sentinel* again used the occasion to attack Fagan personally:

> Apparently Dr. Fagan has an idea he is running the country and can do as he pleases...This sanatorium business may be very entertaining to Dr. Fagan but Kamloops doesn't want it and the sooner the provincial board of health realise this fact the better.[24]

By the time the twenty-five member delegation of the Anti-Sanitarium (in Kamloops) League, led by chairman M.S. Wade, appeared before the city council in late August, not a voice to the contrary was to be heard locally. Consequently, city council unanimously endorsed the petition the league proposed to send to the provincial government. Indeed, it would have been awkward to have done otherwise. The league included most of the prominent members of the local business community, three medical doctors and a minister of religion, all of the local hotel and boarding house operators, and boasted on its executive cattleman Pat Burns, Senator Hewitt Bostock, MP George McCormick and Kamloops mayor J.R. Michell.

Ironically, the same meeting of city council agreed to post copies of a notice, just received from Fagan, to discourage spitting in public places. The petition they then endorsed advanced the arguments that the children of Kamloops needed to be protected against contagion, and that "the town would be overrun by the overflow of the sick, which would be a serious detriment to its inhabitants and their general prosperity." In what must stand as the only instance when the local booster community consciously drew attention to the terrible wind and dust that "constantly" prevailed at Kamloops, the petition pointed out that other more isolated sites existed throughout the dry belt. It drew particular attention to John Shields' offer of ten acres near Ashcroft "with free electric light, water and telephone service." The petitioners concluded that they were strongly opposed to any "means of attracting consumptives to or within 25 miles of the City of Kamloops."[25]

The modern term for this kind of attitude is nimbyism, derived from the expression "Not in my back yard!". It can rarely have found an expression purer than in the position taken by the Anti-Sanitarium (in Kamloops) League. Yet, to a great extent, the attempt to establish a provincial sanatorium had become a tale of two cities, each seeking the same thing. The philanthropic, medical and political establishments, centred in Victoria, desired to bring to British Columbia the benefits of modern medicine. They argued that this should reasonably be expected by the people of a progressive province. Though they differed in many respects, the various Victoria interests certainly agreed that, if a sanatorium was to be built, it should not be located in the populated regions of the lower mainland and Vancouver Island. The prevailing medical opinion favouring dry climates for the treatment of pulmonary conditions pointed conveniently to smaller, more distant interior centres such as Kamloops as the best possible locations. The reaction of the community of Kamloops may have found its expression in a less sophisticated manner, but it was essentially the same as that taken by the leaders of public opinion in Victoria. Build it; but build it elsewhere.

Chapter Notes

1 *Muskoka Sun*, 3 August 1989, pp. 50-51.
2 National Library of Canada, *Second Annual Report of the National Sanitarium Association*, 1898-1899. Differing spellings of sanatorium/sanitarium/sanitorium present an awkward point. Spellings used by historical organizations and institutions have been followed here.
3 E. Furrer, T.W. Lambert, et. al., "General Statistics and Other Information Regarding the Suitability of Kamloops as a Health Resort." (Kamloops, n.d.)
4 Katharine Avis Pumphrey, "Tuberculosis Control in British Columbia," (University of Chicago, 1946, unpublished MA thesis) p. 1.
5 *Inland Sentinel*, 1 March 1895, p. 4.
6 *Inland Sentinel*, 28 February 1896, p. 3.
7 *Inland Sentinel*, 16 May 1899, p. 4.
8 R.E. Gosnell, *A History of British Columbia*, 1906, pp. 559-60.
9 *Inland Sentinel*, 29 January 1901, p. 2.
10 British Columbia Medical Association Archives, J.H. MacDermot Papers, Box 1, file 3.
11 National Archives of Canada, Records of the Canadian Tuberculosis Association, MG 28, I75, volumes 13/14, Appendix I (b).
12 *Kamloops Standard*, 7 March 1901, p. 1.
13 *Kamloops Standard*, 31 January 1902, p. 4.
14 *Kamloops Standard*, 7 February 1901, p. 4; 14 February 1901, p. 4.
15 *Kamloops Standard*, 14 March 1901, p. 2.
16 Georgina Feldberg, *Disease and Class* (New Brunswick, New Jersey, 1995) p. 84.
17 *Kamloops Standard*, 21 February 1901, p. 4.
18 British Columbia *Sessional Papers* 1903, Report of the Provincial Board of Health, pp. J34 and J42. The site was most likely at the east foot of what is today known as Batchelor Hill.
19 NAC, MG 28 I75, volume 11, file 83.
20 *Inland Sentinel*, 30 April 1903, p. 2.
21 *Vancouver Province*, 2 May 1904, p. 5, and *Vancouver Daily News-Advertiser*, 3 May 1904, p. 7.
22 *Kamloops Standard*, 13 August 1904, p. 1.
23 *Vancouver Province*, 11 August 1904, p. 1.
24 *Inland Sentinel*, 9 August 1904, p. 2.
25 BCARS, GR 429, Box 11, file 5, 2970/04. It should be noted that the reaction of Kamloops was by no means unique. In 1908, residents of London, Ontario opposed the opening of a local sanatorium because of the same health concerns and fears of declining property values. In 1908, one member of London City Council said if it were built, "London would become the dumping ground for all consumptives" in western Ontario. See J.T.H. Connor, *A Heritage of Healing* (London, Ontario: 1990, p. 14.) The Queen Alexandra Sanatorium was opened in London in April 1910 by Governor General Earl Grey.

Doctor Fagan's Crusade

Doctor Charles Fagan continued to combine his public appointment and his private campaign. As the province's sole medical health officer, Fagan was secretary to the Provincial Board of Health. After its reorganization in 1899, the Provincial Board of Health wielded extensive powers and was essentially comprised of the lieutenant governor in council. Fagan, therefore, always had the ear of the government, and, according to one medical historian, functioned very much as a chief executive officer. In matters pertaining to health, Fagan's influence was comparable to that of a cabinet member.[1]

Fagan, therefore, was clearly the most influential medical practitioner in British Columbia. His position as medical health officer made him, practically speaking, solely responsible for public health of the non-Native population of a huge geographic area. His recommendations to the Provincial Board of Health were always seriously considered and his suggestions to local doctors were often interpreted as government directives. Provincial regulations covering sanitation in fish canneries, milk preparation and slaughterhouses in the first decade of this century all owe their origins to Fagan and all are suggestive of the growing involvement of government in matters of health.

Fagan and the government agreed that it was appropriate to introduce measures to combat the number-one killer in the province: tuberculosis. Regulations adopted in November 1901 made tuberculosis a reportable disease for the first time in British Columbia. Doctors, teachers, homeowners and hospital supervisors were required by law to report suspected cases to local health officers. At the same time, spitting in public buildings and on tramways was made a summary offence.[2] The Provincial Board of Health was pleased to send its medical health officer to the founding convention of the antituberculous organization being formed by the Canadian Medical Association in Ottawa in February 1901. Fagan was an active participant at the convention and spoke to delegates on the need to reform fashion in women's clothing in the interests of fighting tuberculosis. He argued that the bacillus could remain undisturbed in dust in city streets until:

> ...Miss Fashion comes along, and with an energy worthy of a better cause, sweeps up with her trailing skirt the peaceful bacillus to be inspired by some unfortunate...Miss Fashion does not think she is cruel but by her actions kills thousands.

With characteristic optimism, Fagan concluded: "I refuse to believe that fashion will win against humanity."[3]

Fagan returned to British Columbia as an executive member of the Canadian Association for the Prevention of Consumption and Other Forms of Tuberculosis. He was convinced that it was the proper role of government to educate the public in preventative measures and to provide care for the victims of the disease. Fagan always maintained that a "policy of drift" was indefensible in an "age of progress and knowledge," and he did not hesitate to press upon the provincial government the need for action.[4] By the end of the year, he formally recommended to the attorney general that two sanatoria should be built with government assistance—one for incipient cases and one for advanced cases. He explained the necessity of two institutions, arguing that it would be injurious to the recovery of incipient cases to witness the inevitable deaths of those in advanced stages of the disease. He also provided considerable detail about the site requirements, noting there must be pure air free from dust and moisture, no great temperature changes, and above all "a complete freedom from north and northwest winds."[5]

Fagan also turned his attention to public education by writing "in the simplest way" a circular to accompany the new tuberculosis regulations in November 1901. The four pages of description and instruction provide a full summary of his own perceptions of the disease that had become his adversary and of the methods of treatment available. The pamphlet explained how to create effective disinfecting solutions, and provided detailed advice for victims, attendants, and the public. It invited those who feared they were suffering from the disease to send, preferably under a doctor's guidance, carefully corked bottles containing their sputum to the provincial bacteriological laboratory in Victoria for analysis. There would be no charge to the senders.[6] Every doctor, clergyman, and teacher in British Columbia received a copy of the pamphlet, forty thousand copies of which were distributed.

If Fagan had good reason to be satisfied with the provincial government's support of his educational and preventative measures, he became increasingly frustrated by its inaction concerning treatment. The sympathetic hearing and private assurances of support he received from individual members of the government convinced him that the responsibility for building and operating a tuberculosis sanatorium would soon be accepted by the province. Speculation that an announcement was forthcoming occasionally appeared in newspapers, but the announcement never came. The realization that no government action would occur without public pressure led to the formation of the British Columbia Anti-Tuberculosis Society in January 1904. The desire on the part of the government to see the matter dealt with by private philanthropy also helps to explain the overwhelming support individual politicians extended to the new organization.

Fagan's disappointments were not all derived from the provincial government. As a member of the Committee on Preventative Measures and on Sanatoria, (formed by the National Association for the Prevention of Consumption and other Forms of Tuberculosis), Fagan made a presentation to Prime Minister Wilfrid Laurier during the annual meeting in Ottawa in April 1904. The association had taken the position that the fight against tuberculosis must be seen as a matter of national concern and could not be left to the limited resources of provincial governments alone. Fagan told the prime minister quite bluntly: "I feel confident we will not appeal to our country's governors in vain to right such a condition, and I also feel certain they will not plead the hard and fast lines of the British North America Act as a reply."[7]

The delegation left the meeting well pleased with Laurier's apparent interest in their cause. Within the next year, resolutions favouring federal action were passed by both the House of Commons and the Senate, and Laurier asked the minister of justice for an opinion on how assistance could be accomplished. However, by the time of the annual meeting of 1905, nothing had been achieved and the association called for a royal commission to investigate how to deal with tuberculosis. However, no such commission was appointed and nothing further was done because the creation of the provinces of Alberta and Saskatchewan occupied the paramount position on the government's agenda at the time. The federal government's position was essentially the same as that of the government of British Columbia: it was sympathetic, but unwilling to act.

Added to these disappointments was the knowledge that the fundraising efforts of the fledgling British Columbia Anti-Tuberculosis Society had met with only limited success. Avoiding as much as possible discussion of the question of a specific site, the society attempted at every opportunity to bring before the public the question of antituberculous work and the need for a sanatorium. Particularly in Vancouver and Victoria, lectures by medical officials and visiting celebrities were accompanied by appeals for funds. Though the pledges of $5,000 each from the Canadian Pacific Railway and the provincial government were well publicized, only $2,000 in addition was raised from the public during the first two years of the society's existence.

It was, therefore, a sadder but wiser Doctor Fagan who attended the annual meeting of the national organization in Ottawa in late March 1906. He pointed to the need for branch societies to raise funds for the maintenance of an institution once built. Only then, he argued, could businesses and governments confidently contribute to a building fund. He caused a considerable stir amongst delegates by declaring that after five years of existence, the association could not point to any achievement or reduction in mortality rates from tuberculosis. He also admitted, sadly, that in British Columbia his forty thousand informational circulars had been almost completely ignored. "Anything official coming to the public ear does not enter the brain," he remarked.[8]

Fagan must have been further dismayed when he noted that amongst those attending the conference for the first time was Senator Hewitt Bostock, founding member and figurehead of the Anti-Sanitarium (in Kamloops) League founded two years earlier. Though Bostock did not formally present the views of the league, he did rise to address the delegates "on behalf of British Columbia's dry belt" during a discussion of anti-spitting by-laws. He stated that tubercular sputum quickly dried up in such a climate and was "blown about everywhere" by the winds infecting otherwise healthy people. He regretted that the city of Kamloops had no anti-spitting by-law, and urged delegates to pressure provincial governments to compel municipalities to control spitting. The argument was consistent with the views of the league and was clearly calculated to deflect the meeting from consideration of sanatorium treatment.

Fagan would certainly have enjoyed telling the senator he was evidently unaware of existing regulations in the province that he had been appointed to represent in the Senate. He rose to say that in British Columbia the provincial government had approved anti-spitting regulations in 1901, that nearly all municipalities (including Kamloops) had since complied, and that he had personally fined many individuals for breaking those local by-laws. Fagan left Ottawa in a more optimistic mood, declaring in his final statement to the association that the British Columbia organization was "right in the heart of it" and was determined "to have something done."

Chapter Notes

1 A.S. Monro, The Medical History of British Columbia, *Canadian Medical Association Journal*, 1932, p. 37.
2 British Columbia *Sessional Papers* 1902, Report of the Provincial Board of Health, pp. 778-80.
3 National Archives of Canada (NAC), MG 28 I 75, Records of the Canadian Tuberculosis Association, volumes 13/14, Correspondence.
4 NAC, MG 28 I 75, volume VI, file 6, British Columbia Anti-Tuberculosis Society: "A Summary of the Work Accomplished," p. 3.
5 British Columbia *Sessional Papers* 1902, Report of the Provincial Board of Health, p. 775.
6 NAC MG 28 I 75, volume VI, file 6, "Tuberculosis: Instructions and Suggestions" (Victoria, 1901).
7 NAC MG 28 I 75, Records of the Canadian Tuberculosis Association, volumes 13/14, Appendix I (b).
8 NAC, MG 28 I 75, volume 23, Canadian Association for the Prevention of Consumption and Other Forms of Tuberculosis. Transactions of the Sixth Annual Convention held at Ottawa, 28-29 March 1906, p. 8.

The Sanatorium Established: 1906-07

In Kamloops, after the conversion of the Inland Board of Trade to its view, the Anti-Sanitarium League lapsed into inactivity. With both newspapers and the business community on side, a separate organization hardly seemed necessary. Proponents of a local sanatorium were few, and when Dr. Procter accepted an appointment as CPR physician in Vancouver in April 1905, the British Columbia Anti-Tuberculosis Society lost its most vocal supporter in Kamloops. Perhaps sensing an advantage, the Inland Board of Trade invited Fagan to address a meeting in Kamloops in July. However, the meeting became a public relations triumph for Dr. Fagan. He assured those present that if Kamloops was serious about its objections to a sanatorium being located within city boundaries, those wishes would be respected. An editorial in the previously hostile *Kamloops Standard* expressed satisfaction that other locations in the dry belt were under consideration and concluded that Kamloops had nothing to fear.[1] From this time forward, the *Standard* became a staunch supporter of the Anti-Tuberculosis Society.

To add to the public success, on the same visit Fagan recruited one of the most influential men in Kamloops as a member of the society. Marsh Gordon had arrived in Kamloops thirty years earlier seeking a cure for his asthma. He had long been active with the Board of Trade and in civic politics, but he had not been a signatory to the petition of the Anti-Sanitarium (in Kamloops) League the previous year. In 1905, he was elected mayor of the city and president of the Inland Board of Trade, and in January 1906, he was re-elected mayor.

However, opposition to the location of a sanatorium within or anywhere near Kamloops remained strong. The Board of Trade and the *Inland Sentinel* newspaper, with sanatorium opponent M.S. Wade as its new owner and editor, continued forcefully to represent the contrary position. In May 1906, the Board of Trade advised the Anti-Tuberculosis Society that it would support the founding of a sanatorium in British Columbia only if it were located more than fifteen miles from the city of Kamloops. The Board of Trade invited Fagan to respond by addressing another public meeting in Kamloops, knowing that Fagan's agreement to that principle would signal a complete victory for the opponents of a local sanatorium.

Again Fagan accepted the invitation, and again he satisfied the majority of his listeners. He told the meeting that he never advised his own patients to treat their tuberculosis in Kamloops, as the city was far too dusty and windy. He made it clear, however, that Kamloops Lake had become the society's preferred location, and that a sanatorium located five miles east of Savona near Six Mile Point was a strong possibility. The meeting passed one resolution to support the founding of a sanatorium "near but not in" Kamloops, and another to encourage the formation of a local branch of the Anti-Tuberculosis Society. Nearly satisfied, the Board of Trade became much less vocal about the matter. The *Sentinel*, on the other hand, continued to snipe. It soon reported and regretted the death near Savona of a young Englishman suffering from tuberculosis, but could not resist adding that he had been sent there by Fagan "as a test case."

Outside Kamloops, the issue of sanatorium location generated little comment. After its much-publicized founding in 1904, the British Columbia Anti-Tuberculosis Society had set about its business with both energy and enthusiasm. However, it was an enthusiasm the public was reluctant to embrace. The society was very much centred in Victoria. Its postal address was given as the Government Buildings and it had solid support in the political and philanthropic communities of the city. Frequent events, such as the concert by the Margherita Mandolin Club, raised money and created publicity for the society in the city. Fagan resided in Victoria and all the society's meetings were held there. But apart from some token membership in the Vancouver area, the society barely existed outside Victoria. It became apparent, therefore, that further effort in publicity and fundraising would be necessary if the dream of a provincial sanatorium was to become reality.

Immediately upon Fagan's return from the Ottawa convention of 1906, decisions were made to extend the organization of the society beyond its narrow Victoria base and to launch a major fundraising effort. The means selected to achieve this goal was the formation of local auxiliary societies throughout the province. The auxiliaries would provide the parent society with both a presence and an organization outside the Victoria area, and would demonstrate to government that support for the movement was widespread. They would also raise money for maintenance costs once the proposed sanatorium was finally built. As Fagan had remarked previously, only after the society had proven its ability to operate a sanatorium could it confidently approach the business community for contributions to the building fund. Wherever his duties as medical health officer took him during the next twelve months, Fagan arranged public meetings. The purpose of the gatherings was to recruit local members and to encourage the formation of branch societies. In a series of motivational speeches, Fagan made it clear that this charitable work was a field the women of each community should claim as their own.[2]

The first auxiliary was formed in Victoria in the summer of 1906, establishing the pattern of other auxiliaries that soon would follow. Comprised largely of the wives and daughters of locally prominent political, professional, and business figures, the Victoria auxiliary was proud to have Mrs. James Dunsmuir, wife of the newly appointed lieutenant-governor, as its honorary president. Within two years, the large membership in the Victoria branch society permitted a division into a senior society for married women and a junior society for unmarried women. Auxiliaries formed in other centres could not equal the Victoria branch in either numbers or symbolism. However, like the Victoria branch, their membership was entirely female and was drawn almost exclusively from the same social classes. By the end of 1907, ten branches of the British Columbia Anti-Tuberculosis Society had been formed throughout the province.

In September 1906, the fundraising campaign was officially launched with Fagan's announcement that Lieutenant-Governor James Dunsmuir had personally pledged to donate $10,000 as soon as $50,000 could be raised from other sources. The *Kamloops Standard*, as if to atone for its earlier opposition, resorted to hyperbole in announcing the campaign. The newspaper urged its readers to contribute, stating that to stand idly by any longer would be "tantamount to something worse than race suicide."[3] Encouraged by the growing number of auxiliaries and by donations over the winter of 1906-07, the society concluded that the time for action had arrived. Delegates from organizations and municipalities from throughout the province were invited to attend the fourth annual meeting of the British Columbia Anti-Tuberculosis Society to be held at city hall in Victoria in early April 1907. Mayor Marsh Gordon represented Kamloops at the request of the city council, attending what the *Sentinel* derisively described as the society's "annual spouting bee."[4]

The meeting agreed that $100,000 would be necessary to build an effective sanatorium, but was pleased to note that donations—apart from Dunsmuir's—had reached $38,000, and cheered Fagan's prediction that a further $12,000 could be raised within a month. Delegates learned that the auxiliary societies throughout the province had raised an additional $4,000 to pay for the maintenance of indigent patients at the proposed sanatorium. Providing further encouragement was the announcement that the federal government had promised to donate up to 400 acres of Crown land at Fish Lake (modern-day Lac Le Jeune) near Kamloops to be used for the treatment of tuberculosis. For the first time, it appeared that the society could count on the active support of both the provincial and federal levels of government in its efforts to provide a care facility for victims of tuberculosis.

The critical moment had arrived. The society officially incorporated itself under provincial statute, adopted a new organizational structure with a complete set of bylaws, and decided it was time to face the serious question of sanatorium location. Fagan expressed the society's gratitude to the federal government for its generosity, noting that Fish Lake would be an ideal site to locate small chalets for the treatment of incipient cases. He added, however, that Fish Lake could not be the location of the main treatment facility due to its high elevation. The meeting then enthusiastically appointed a committee that included Dr. Fagan, Dr. William Stephen, and Marsh Gordon to travel through the dry belt to investigate a number of prospective properties.

If most members of the British Columbia Anti-Tuberculosis Society looked forward to the challenge eagerly, some had their reservations. The society had recently employed two nurses, treating patients in five tents in Victoria and, occasionally, in a shack at Six Mile Point near Savona. It would create a much greater burden of responsibility to build, equip, and operate a sanatorium. Less than half of the $100,000 required to build the sanatorium had been secured, and the question of how much should be spent in site acquisition had not been addressed. In addition, many delegates felt strongly that the society's action in confronting tuberculosis provided a convenience that released the provincial government from its own obligations. One delegate noted that the work of fighting tuberculosis was such that it should be undertaken by the state, but "as the state could not be prevailed upon to undertake it, the action devolved upon the public." He expressed the hope that, later, "the state would do its duty in the matter."[5]

To fulfil their duties, the site selection committee travelled to the dry belt in early July. The first property considered was the Lyons ranch at North Bend in the Fraser Canyon. The asking price of $12,000 was judged far too high, though the committee considered that at a much-reduced price the ranch could perhaps be the site of a second sanatorium for advanced consumptives at a future date. Apparently not even pausing to consider the property offered by John Shields near Ashcroft, the committee stopped next at Savona. There they were met, at the request of Marsh Gordon, by Kamloops council member John Robinson who agreed to conduct them to the several locations being considered. On 8 July, the committee was taken by boat to six separate sites on Kamloops Lake, including the location near Six Mile Point, which was considered the most likely choice. But at each site, most of which were on the lake's south shore, considerations such as exposure, prevailing winds or water supply were found to a greater or lesser extent to be unsatisfactory. Robinson then suggested a visit to a property at Tranquille, some thirteen kilometres west of Kamloops on the north shore of Kamloops Lake. This was the location that had so impressed William Van Horne and Thomas Roddick in 1899. Familiar with the site from previous visits, Fagan agreed that the other committee members should see it.

The two extensive ranches located at Tranquille had occasionally accepted as boarders people suffering from mild cases of tuberculosis. The ranch further to the west, owned by Charles Cooney, was not for sale. However, the property owned by William Fortune had been on the market for years. In 1888, the Fortunes sold the ranch to buyers who constructed a fine new eighteen-room house next to the original Fortune ranch house. Subsequently, the new owners failed to meet their financial obligations and the Fortunes reluctantly repossessed the property in 1892. Offered for sale through property agents in Kamloops and New Westminster ever since at a price of $75,000, the ranch had been unable to attract a buyer. Consequently, the Fortunes had informally asked Robinson in April 1907 to act for them in selling the ranch, promising a healthy commission should he be successful. Appalled at the asking price, Robinson nevertheless agreed to try, but he had yet to find a prospective buyer. Curiously, he did not advise the committee that he was a real estate agent.

On the afternoon of the committee's visit, William Fortune was away from the ranch, but Jane Fortune was glad to entertain her unexpected guests. By all accounts a formidable woman, her local nickname "Lady Jane" apparently was more indicative of a strong personality than of refinement. As she served tea, she bluntly asked the committee why they did not purchase her ranch for their sanatorium. In reply, Dr. Fagan spoke for them all when he replied, just as bluntly: "Oh, you want too much." Yet the committee members all admitted they were impressed by the 560-acre ranch with its southern exposure, its mile of lake frontage, its extensive leased grazing lands, and the "absolute protection" afforded by neighbouring mountains against northerly winds. As they toured the property, they began to consider, apparently for the first time, not only the issues of sanatorium location, but also the advantages of an assured food supply for the institution. Dr. Fagan did not accompany the other committee members as they walked about the property. Instead, he chatted with Jane Fortune, who took the opportunity to offer him $2,000 privately if he could persuade the society to purchase the ranch for $60,000. He declined firmly, but recognized that the property was not as outrageously priced as he had believed.[6]

Continuing on to Kamloops, the committee found itself as featured guests at yet another public meeting called on 11 July to discuss the contentious issue of sanatorium location. Though the meeting at the Kamloops Music and Athletic Association Hall attracted only a small audience, the committee had to contend with the vociferous objections of Kamloops alderman G.D. Brown. Previously, Brown had complained that people throughout the province refused to visit

Kamloops in the belief the hotels were full of consumptives. He had also persuaded council to object to the federal grant at Fish Lake, and he returned to that theme at the meeting. He argued that Fish Lake "was the only place the people of Kamloops had as a pleasure resort and wanted to know how the people of Victoria would take it if Beacon Hill were to be chosen as a sanatorium site." Fagan repeated that the society's intention was to use the Fish Lake site only seasonally and only for patients with mild afflictions. Few Kamloops residents seemed to share Brown's strong views. The *Standard* newspaper, while deploring the poor turnout for the meeting, pointedly editorialized: "From a humanitarian standpoint, from a sanitary standpoint, in fact from any standpoint the result will be a benefit to Kamloops, and the puerile, selfish and short-sighted efforts to place obstacles in the way of the sanatorium directors should cease."[7] The *Sentinel* commented only briefly, noting that "the sanitarium chestnut" had been discussed at a poorly attended meeting.

While in Kamloops, Dr. Stephen visited the power house with John Robinson to make enquiries about the costs of installing and operating a pumping station as would be required at most of the Kamloops Lake locations. The visit confirmed that these costs would be substantial. The committee was convinced that the water supplied by Tranquille Creek at the Fortune ranch would allow the society to avoid the cost of installing a pumping station, and believed that the Fortunes would accept a much lower sum than the $75,000 listed price. They returned to Tranquille to make an offer subject to the approval of the society's board of directors. William and Jane Fortune accepted $58,000 and agreed to become life governors of the British Columbia Anti-Tuberculosis Society by returning $1,000 of the purchase price to the society. After a day trip to inspect Crown lands at Fish Lake, the committee returned to the coast.

The committee's report and recommendations were submitted to the board on 24 July. The proposed purchase of the Fortune Ranch was controversial because it entailed a financial commitment far greater than anticipated and because it would involve the society in the operation of a ranch, an obligation previously unconsidered by the board. However, persuaded by the force of the report and by the arguments of Dr. Procter and Marsh Gordon, the board accepted the recommendation to acquire the Fortune ranch as the site of the society's sanatorium. Fagan, Gordon, and Stephen were authorized to proceed with arrangements to complete the purchase. All ranch property, buildings, barns, stock, and the rights to lease lands would be acquired for an effective price of $57,000. With insufficient funds to purchase the ranch outright, $25,000 was to be given immediately to the Fortunes, who would hold the balance as a mortgage at five-percent interest. The decision was made to proceed at once to refurbish existing ranch buildings so that the treatment of patients would not have to wait until a new sanatorium building was completed. On 25 July 1907, the board proudly announced the purchase of the Fortune ranch and made public the report of the site selection committee.

The reaction of the Kamloops newspapers was, to some extent, quite predictable. Both printed the entire report of the committee as their lead articles. Applauding the decision, the *Standard* commended the committee members for the wisdom of their choice.

> No more suitable location could be found within the limits of the province than the one at Tranquille, and Kamloops will reap considerable advantage from the establishment which could not have accrued to the city had the location been at a point further down the lake.[8]

But if the sanatorium would be just far enough away in the eyes of its supporters, it would be far too close for its opponents. M.S. Wade at the *Sentinel* insisted that the wishes of Kamloops had been ignored, that the Fortune ranch should have been sub-divided into small fruit farms for wealthy families, and that the name Kamloops would necessarily be associated with the sanatorium, "with what result the citizens of the city [would] not be long in discovering to their sorrow." Arguing that the sanatorium had been "foisted upon" Kamloops, Wade concluded:

> With a limited capacity, the sanatorium will be filled to overflowing from all sections of the province, and from without, within a day of its opening. The overflow will abide in Kamloops, a charge upon the public and a menace to the health of its people. That is the

> outcome in a nutshell of Dr. Fagan's labors in the field of humanitarianism.

Not content to let Fagan off so lightly, the newspaper also printed an anonymous "Ode to Fagan" that occupied a full column. Hurriedly written, the poem is distinguished only by the sarcasm and bitterness it directs at its unfortunate subject.[9]

If these personal attacks ruffled Dr. Fagan, he made no public response. Undoubtedly as an employee of the provincial government he was under some constraint, even when he was acting privately as a member of the Anti-Tuberculosis Society and even when he was attacked personally. However, it is likely that he simply had no time even to contemplate a battle with his critics in Kamloops. With the site of the sanatorium decided at last, the work of the Anti-Tuberculosis Society began in earnest, and no one took that work more seriously than Dr. Fagan. He was on the committee responsible for completing the agreement for sale, and he was in charge of the search for a suitable medical superintendent and matron. He decided to use his vacation from his duties as medical health officer in October to oversee personally the many preparations necessary to receive the society's first patients at the Fortune ranch. At the same time, an outbreak of smallpox in the Kootenays interrupted his vacation and required his official attention.

At Tranquille, the old Fortune ranch house and the newer and larger adjacent building—both on stone foundations—were thought to be serviceable, and renovations were begun. However, the buildings required greater attention than originally anticipated. At night, the walls in the kitchen seemed to be moving. Closer examination showed that an infestation of cockroaches was housed between layers of wallpaper. Several old hogsheads were found to contain Mrs. Fortune's locally famous plum wine, but the surface of each was covered with "a good layer of flies, bugs, mosquitoes and other repulsive debris." The plum wine was dumped into Kamloops Lake. When furniture coverings had become old or dirty, Jane Fortune apparently had been in the habit of simply adding a new layer of covering. The first medical superintendent of the sanatorium, in a subsequent memoir, described this encounter between Dr. Fagan and Jane Fortune:

> Some of the chairs had six layers and certainly were not sanitary. Dr. Fagan decided to have these burnt up; when Mrs. Fortune saw him there was a battle royal. He told her that the chairs and furniture were loaded with germs and had a lot of tubercle bacilli in them. She said she had lived there for thirty years and had never seen any.[10]

The furniture was burned, as were all the curtains and carpets. By the time the first patients arrived at the end of November, the buildings had been thoroughly cleaned and painted, some walls had been removed, and a new septic system and several fireplaces had been installed. The cost of the preparations, at $4,000, was higher than anticipated.[11]

The search for a superintendent had begun even before the site selection committee travelled to the interior, but the cash-strapped society ran into difficulties immediately. It is unlikely that their claim to have received thirty applications for the position can be believed. The search for the right man was extended to eastern Canada, the United States, and even to Germany. The chief physician at a New York State sanatorium replied to Fagan's enquiry thus:

> I have not on my staff at present any physician who would care to accept the appointment in your proposed institution with the responsibilities and duties involved at anything like the remuneration which you propose to allow, and cannot therefore assist you in your present undertaking.[12]

By mid-October, with the first patients scheduled to arrive at month's end, a medical superintendent had yet to be appointed. At that time, Fagan, as chief examiner on the provincial medical examinations board, made the acquaintance of Robert Washington Irving, a young doctor from Ontario seeking accreditation in British Columbia. Learning that Irving had some experience at the sanatorium in Gravenhurst, Fagan asked if he would be interested in going up to Kamloops to open the new sanatorium at Tranquille. Dr. Irving agreed. At the board of directors meeting on 31 October, he was appointed as temporary medical superintendent for a period of six months, after which time the board expected to make a permanent appointment. At the same meeting of the board, Jean Matheson of Qu'Appelle in Saskatchewan, was appointed matron. A former matron at Royal Inland Hospital, Matheson had returned to Saskatchewan in 1905, but wrote to Fagan applying for the position at Tranquille in early October 1906.[13]

Irving arrived in Kamloops in the early hours of the morning on 10 November 1907. He was taken to the Leland Hotel, then under construction, where, as he later recalled, he "spent the rest of the night trying to keep warm." When he was waiting for Jean Matheson to arrive later the same morning, Irving found himself reflecting that Kamloops—with its dust and wind and blowing sagebrush—looked a dreary sight indeed. They were met by W.W. Shaw of Shuswap, who had been engaged as farm manager in mid-summer. Together for the first time as their horse-drawn carriage took them towards Tranquille, the three supervisors—superintendent, matron, and farm manager—undoubtedly discussed and contemplated the magnitude of the responsibilities they had taken on. In just a matter of days, the sanatorium would be open for business.

Chapter Notes

1 *Kamloops Standard*, 15 July 1905, pp. 1 and 4.
2 National Archives of Canada, MG 28, I 75, volume VI, file 6, British Columbia Anti-Tuberculosis Society: "A Summary of the Work Accomplished," p. 2.
3 *Kamloops Standard*, 20 October 1906, p. 8.
4 *Inland Sentinel*, 5 April 1907, p. 1.
5 University of British Columbia (UBC), Records of the British Columbia Anti-Tuberculosis Society, Court of Governors Book, pp. 31-33.
6 *Kamloops Standard*, 9 November 1907, p. 1; Inland Sentinel, 8 November 1907, p. 1 and p. 5.
7 *Kamloops Standard*, 13 July 1907, p. 1 and p. 4.
8 *Kamloops Standard*, 27 July 1907, p. 4.
9 *Inland Sentinel*, 26 July 1907, pp. 2-3.
10 British Columbia Archives and Records Service (BCARS), GR 2866, box 1, file 1, Robert Irving, "The Early Days of Tranquille Sanatorium."
11 BCARS, Additional MSS 1916, Records of the British Columbia Anti-Tuberculosis Society, Letter Book, p. 21.
12 Kamloops Museum and Archives, Tranquille Sanatorium files.
13 UBC, Records of the British Columbia Anti-Tuberculosis Society, Minute Book of the Board of Directors, p. 8.

Growing Pains: 1907-1910

On 28 November, a group of seven tubercular patients from the lower mainland and Vancouver Island arrived in Kamloops. They were under the care of Mrs. Clark, the first nurse to be employed at the sanatorium. Previously with the Victorian Order of Nurses in Vancouver, she was instructed to meet three other patients at Kamloops and to conduct the entire group to Tranquille immediately. The small party was "jolted out the nine miles from Kamloops by horse-drawn stage" and with their arrival, the Tranquille Sanatorium declared itself officially open. A Union Jack was hoisted on the flagstaff of the reconstructed larger ranch house, and Fagan cabled Irving: "Congratulations, and may success attend all your efforts." Canada's seventh sanatorium—the first west of Ontario—was open for business.

It was the end of a difficult month. Preparation of the old Fortune ranch buildings and awkward legal matters had fully occupied the society, especially its energetic secretary Dr. Fagan. He and Dr. Stephen were required to attend the Kamloops courthouse on 6 November to give evidence in a civil action suit brought by John Robinson against William Fortune. Robinson insisted he was owed a commission of $1,000 on the sale of the ranch to the Anti-Tuberculosis Society; William and Jane Fortune insisted no such obligation had been incurred. The proceedings attracted much local interest and the courthouse was packed. Testimony revealed more than Robinson's failure to disclose his occupation and Jane Fortune's private offer to Dr. Fagan. Jane Fortune had offered $25 to settle the matter and a shouting match occurred with an insulted John Robinson. Testimony revealed that the listing property agents had agreed to forego commission because the sale was to a charitable organization, and that the Anti-Tuberculosis Society was surprised that Robinson was insisting on a commission. When the court, quite unexpectedly, decided completely in favour of Robinson, William Fortune declared he would seek $1,000 as full compensation from the society.

On 7 November, Fagan was again at Tranquille, on a final "tour of inspection" to ensure all was in readiness to receive the first patients. However, legal matters continued to demand attention. When Fagan and Marsh Gordon attended the law offices of Frederick Fulton on 8 November to sign final papers relating to the ranch purchase, they were advised of further complications. Fortune did not possess a survey to verify the location of the dividing line between his property and the Cooney ranch. Secondly, forty acres of land that Fortune had agreed to sell to the society was occupied and claimed by a Chinese settler. Nothing would be signed until these matters were settled, and much unpleasantness resulted between the Fortunes and the Anti-Tuberculosis Society. However, neither party seriously considered withdrawing from the real estate transaction. The Fortunes were preparing for an extended visit to Britain, and the society had no desire to renew the controversial process of site selection.

With the sanatorium an established fact, opposition within Kamloops continued to diminish. The resolution of May 1906 calling for the formation of a local branch society in Kamloops had not achieved the desired result. But with the presence of Dr. Fagan in the city undoubtedly providing further encouragement, the British Columbia Anti-Tuberculosis Society saw the formation of its tenth auxiliary in early November 1907. On the same day of Fagan's visit to the Fulton law offices, the Kamloops Ladies Auxiliary officially began its life with Mrs. Marsh Gordon as president and Isabel Costley as secretary. As its first major fundraising event, the auxiliary hosted a "Calico Ball" at the Kamloops Musical and Athletic Association Hall on 1 January 1908, and held its first annual meeting in council chambers on 7 January. Both the local and provincial organizations were cheered by the results of the municipal election a few days later. The sanatorium was an issue in the campaign, but did not determine the outcome. Anti-Tuberculosis Society supporter John Robinson, campaigning primarily to relocate the Kamloops Indian Band away from the city, easily defeated sanatorium opponent G.D. Brown in the mayoralty contest. By early December, just a week after it opened, the sanatorium reached its full capacity with sixteen patients in residence. One of the sixteen was Annie Forest—the first admission from the city of Kamloops.

At Irving's request, Fagan and Stephen visited again in January to investigate the capacity of the ranch houses and transportation difficulties. Because of their visit, a motor launch was purchased for sanatorium use at a cost of $700, and the society agreed to supply a horse for the medical superintendent and to pay for its upkeep. By mid-March, with funds collected by the Vancouver auxiliary, two tent cottages were built for ambulatory male patients. Capacity thereby increased to twenty-two patients and plans for two more small cottages would soon increase the number of patients to twenty-six. Modest attempts to emulate the cottage system at Saranac, the Tranquille cottages were located adjacent to the old ranch house facing the lake. Intended as temporary accommodation, the cottages would be used for fifteen years and were quickly dubbed "the shacks" by patients. Irving was accommodated in the two-room house that had been moved across the lake from Six Mile Point, while Jean Matheson occupied one of the rooms in the renovated Fortune ranch house.

However, these arrangements were regarded as no more than temporary. In March 1908, at its first official meeting, the Court of Governors optimistically decided to press forward. Despite an insufficiency of funds, the directors were authorized "to proceed with the many buildings in connection with the Sanatorium for Incipient Consumptives, and the Ranch connected therewith."[1] The first building, of course, would be the sanatorium itself. Fagan and others had given much thought to the advantages and disadvantages of various models. Should the German system of a single building be adopted, or would the more expensive American cottage system with its "home-like influence" be preferable? The society's financial situation pointed to the single-building option. Fagan provided photographs and illustrations of institutions from all over the world, urging that the model of British designer Dr. Latham be modified to suit the society's purpose and budget. Architect W.T. Dalton of the lower mainland firm Dalton and Eveleigh was asked to design a suitable building. He accepted the commission, and the society immediately sent him to study the construction of existing sanatoria in eastern Canada and New England.

Irving was pleased that the isolated location discouraged patients from making frequent trips to Kamloops. He also noted other advantages: "Those who are accustomed to take periodically too much alcoholic stimulants have that temptation removed, and they are not annoyed by too frequent visitors."[2] He remarked that the isolation made it difficult to secure an all-white workforce, but that it was his intention to do so. Whether Irving was expressing a personal opinion or whether he was responding to British Columbia's prevalent anti-Asiatic prejudices is uncertain. In the meantime, the facility continued to be served by two Chinese cooks and a Chinese laundryman.

By the spring of 1908, Dr. Irving was looking forward to discharging the first cured patients. However, expressing a note of concern that was to occupy successive sanatorium administrators for decades, he told a local newspaper that the majority of patients at the sanatorium were advanced cases for whom little could be done. Though it was the intention of the British Columbia Anti-Tuberculosis Society to offer care at Tranquille only to incipient cases, Irving said it was in the interests of the public to provide the terminally ill "with the benefit of a few weeks treatment."[3]

The sanatorium experienced an unpleasant public controversy in April when Dr. Irving expelled a patient for insubordination. The former patient quickly contacted Dr. Stephen in New Westminster alleging that the quality of food was poor, that an excessive delay occurred in the removal of a dead body, and that Irving disdained him as a non-paying patient. The *Vancouver Province* published his letter outlining the complaints.[4] Fagan and four other members of the board of directors wasted no time in travelling to Tranquille to investigate. They found all the complaints to be without substance, but they insisted that, in future, all such situations were to be handled by the board and not by the medical superintendent.

The society did agree that Irving should have the assistance of a business manager, and in the late spring, A.M. Tyrrell came out from Gravenhurst to act as bursar. However, he arrived before his accommodation was ready and he was placed in one of the tent cottages at a time when the mosquitoes were at their worst. Irving would later recall that Tyrrell was bitten all over and that the bulls in the orchard, themselves tormented by the mosquitoes, ran around Tyrrell's tent cottage bawling all night. For protection, Irving then bought “all the cheesecloth there was in Kamloops.”[5] Later that summer, the board also agreed to build a house for the use of the medical superintendent and to raise the matron's monthly salary to $60. Irving's request was granted for a two-month leave in September and October to attend the international symposium on tuberculosis in Washington, D.C.

In the summer of 1908, the society suffered a surprising setback at the hands of the federal government. In place of the proposed grant of land at Fish Lake, the society apparently requested the grant of a portion of the lease lands adjacent to the sanatorium ranch. At Shaw's suggestion, the ranch had been named Alexandra Ranch in honour of the queen, and in a letter to Frank Oliver, minister of the interior, Fagan noted that the ranch operation was central to the success of the institution. Production of their own food supply would ensure its purity and would allow the sanatorium to be more self-sufficient. Furthermore, if the Alexandra Ranch could produce surpluses as anticipated, the sale of those surpluses would provide income to support the operation of the sanatorium itself. Letters in support of the request were sent by Fagan to Laurier and to all British Columbia's senators and MPs. In July, the society was shocked when it was informed that, because it was going into “cattle ranching and general farming on a large scale” for profit, it could not be viewed as a purely philanthropic organization. Therefore, it would not receive a land grant. The Fish Lake proposal was not revived, and the society was forced to recognize it would receive no more than verbal support from Ottawa.[6]

With the benefit of his eastern excursion to draw upon, Dalton submitted architectural plans for a modern sanatorium to the board during the summer. The plans, a modified version of Latham's King's Hospital in London, called for extensive verandahs and balconies. Tenders were invited for the construction of a building it was estimated would cost $80,000. With the submission of the surprisingly low bid of $65,000, the Vancouver construction firm of William O'Dell was awarded the contract. On 14 October 1908, Fagan performed the ceremonial sod turning and work began later that month. The laying of the building's cornerstone by Lieutenant-Governor James Dunsmuir was planned to take place on 11 November. This was a moment long anticipated by members of the Anti-Tuberculosis Society and they intended to use the opportunity well. Dr. Fagan and Dr. Procter arrived early on 10 November to arrange for their expected guests. The lieutenant-governor was to be accompanied by his wife and daughter. Also present would be Mayor Bethune of Vancouver, society president and CPR executive Richard Marpole, John Robinson of Kamloops and former British Columbia premier Charles Semlin.

The sternwheeler *C.R. Lamb* arrived at Tranquille at two o'clock to receive the salute of honour from the Rocky Mountain Rangers. Other guests arrived on the *Silver Stream*. After an extensive speech by Fagan about the history of the movement to establish a sanatorium in British Columbia, the cornerstone was placed over a time capsule. Inside were the minutes of the first meeting of the British Columbia Anti-Tuberculosis Society and a list of its members. A nugget of gold from Tranquille Creek was to be included in the time capsule, but seeking to lead the fundraising campaign by example, Fagan purchased the nugget, writing a cheque in favour of the society. The lieutenant-governor declared the laying of the cornerstone duly accomplished. In Kamloops that evening, a dance, organized by the Kamloops ladies auxiliary and presided over by the vice-regal family, took place at the Kamloops Musical and Athletic Association Hall. Unfortunately, the fifty people aboard the *Silver Stream* were unable to attend what the local newspaper later described as the "brightest social function of the season." Their boat was stuck on a sand bar for eight hours while attempting the return trip from Tranquille.[7]

Despite continuing concern over finances and the disappointment over the lease lands, the year 1908 ended with all seeming well for the Anti-Tuberculosis Society. The status of the sanatorium was enhanced when King Edward VII agreed to add his name to those of the Governor General and the Lieutenant-Governor as a patron of the society. Fagan's personal status was enhanced when he was elected president of the British Columbia Medical Association for 1909. So encouraged was he by the progress achieved that he renewed his attempts to reach the public through his official office. He penned a two-part pamphlet entitled "The Bacillus 'at Home'." The first part, intended for teachers and clergy, provided more statistics than the pamphlet of 1901, quoted the poet Schiller, and appealed more emotionally than previously for support by describing pathetic scenes:

> Infants absorbing death germs with their mother's milk. Parental kisses poisoning the lips of the little ones. Children infected with the class-room dust or snared with fair-seeming sweetmeats from the stall...Belles of the ball-room wearing the dainty things over which some poor sweated woman, perhaps, has coughed her life away...Rich and poor, Dives and Lazarus, linked together, inextricably bound, in the levelling presence of a common curse.

The second part of the pamphlet, for school children and their parents, generally encouraged hygienic habits and listed two dozen admonitions to students with which any teacher could concur. "Don't spit about" headed the list. Yet, the tone of the pamphlet is remarkably optimistic, representing more than anything a call to arms. Fagan clearly envisioned an eventual triumph against "the tuberculosis fiend."[8]

The CPR constructed Tranquille Siding directly across the lake from the sanatorium, specifically so construction materials, coal, and other supplies—some of which were donated by lower mainland firms—could be unloaded there and barged across the lake to Tranquille. In summer, arriving patients were met at Tranquille Siding by Shaw in the new motor launch. Most of the smaller Fortune ranch buildings, including the shell of the old mill, were demolished and O'Dell was beginning the construction of the new building. A telephone connection with Kamloops was established, and many Kamloops merchants signalled their acceptance of the new institution by donating goods and gifts at Christmas. The first (and perhaps only) issue of a publication called the *Tranquille Tattler* was printed and given to the thirty-one patients. Dr. Irving, dressed as Saint Nicholas on Christmas Eve, distributed the more than three hundred gifts the patients had received in the mail.

Care and Controversy

Doctor Irving's previous experience with tuberculosis care was limited. He had been on the medical staff at Gravenhurst for only a few months in 1903 before entering private practice in Ontario for three years. The treatment received by patients at Tranquille was based upon the experience and knowledge he had acquired during his time at Gravenhurst and upon the efforts and abilities of the institution's two nurses. With no days off, the medical staff was available on a twenty-four hour basis, seven days a week. Possessing only a single microscope and a few drugs as his medical supplies, Irving focussed upon a combination of diet, rest, and fresh air as the basis of treatment.

Conventional wisdom at the time insisted that eggs and milk were essential to the successful treatment of tuberculosis, and Shaw immediately began converting ranch production to those ends. The dairy herd was expanded and large chicken coops were constructed to satisfy the demand for one hundred dozen eggs per week. By the end of 1908, the ranch was supplying most of the meat and all the milk required by the sanatorium. But diet alone could not cure the disease. One early patient surprised Irving by consuming two dozen eggs daily. Though he put on weight, his condition worsened, and rest was determined as his best treatment. By the end of the second year of operation, the "extensive and persistent use of raw eggs" was abandoned. Irving reported that after a few weeks of six to eight eggs a day, patients lost their appetite for all food.[9]

One form of therapy came to be known as the refrigeration (or fresh air) treatment. Patients were required to be outdoors from 9 a.m. until 8:30 p.m., even during bitterly cold weather, in the belief that the cold air would stimulate their appetites. Once dried after their daily ice-sponge bath, they were bundled up and seated on the spacious verandahs that had been built onto the old Fortune buildings. Another school of thought held that limited amounts of exercise would contribute to a cure. Fagan assumed that able patients would assist in the work of the Alexandra Ranch, both for their own benefit and for the benefit of the balance sheet of the sanatorium. Beginning in the second year of operations, controlled activity was often prescribed. Irving reported to Fagan towards the end of 1909:

> Work as a medicinal agent has been used in many cases. The results have been pleasing in a majority of cases. This is particularly so in the labouring classes, who are accustomed to manual labour and who have

to be prepared to take up some of the heavier occupations as a means of livelihood after leaving the Sanatorium.[10]

The financial requirements of the institution occupied much of the attention of the society, and these requirements fell into two broad categories: building and maintenance. Despite much effort and publicity, donations to the building fund were disappointing, and just $26,000 remained on hand after paying $25,000 to William Fortune and after renovating the existing buildings. Furthermore, the interest on the mortgage due to the Fortunes—$800, payable twice yearly—was to be drawn from this fund. Fagan was quoted saying only three things were needed to carry out the plans for the sanatorium successfully: "First, money; second, money; third, more money."[11]

Additional donors were found. The editor of the *Victoria Colonist* donated $1,000, thereby becoming a director of the society, and Pat Burns reversed the opposition shown in signing the Anti-Sanitarium (in Kamloops) League petition in 1904. By donating $1,000 in 1908, he, too, became a director. By the end of 1909, just over $135,000 had been pledged. However, the society was frustrated that $18,000 of this amount had not been received. In its third annual report, it admonished its reluctant contributors: "All promises made have in many ways been made public...The withdrawal and the reason should receive the same publicity as was given to the promise." To a very considerable extent, only the support of the provincial government allowed the building programme to proceed. The government pledged (and lived up to its pledges) $5,000 in 1907 and in 1908, $20,000 in 1909 and another $20,000 in 1910. Other contributors included Rossland City Council, the citizens of Ashcroft and Enderby, the Dramatic Club of Revelstoke, and many fraternal organizations and trades unions in the Victoria area.[12]

A portion of the government grant was conditional on the construction of a facility for advanced cases, and the society had certainly not lost sight of its original intention to operate a separate sanatorium for that purpose. Abandoning its earlier preference for the Lyon ranch near Big Bend, in July 1909 the society formally advised the government that the Cooney property adjacent to the Tranquille sanatorium would be ideal and could be purchased for "less than

$70,000."[13] Nothing came of the suggestion and the society quickly realized that the construction of a second facility would be ill advised at a time when the financing of the first was so problematic.

However, the question of patient admissions was a real concern for the society. Intended as a facility for incipient cases only, the existing sanatorium found that, from the very beginning, most patients seeking admission were in an advanced stage of the disease. By 1910, most of the patients admitted to Tranquille had little hope of recovery. The muted hostility of the *Inland Sentinel* could still be heard in its unfortunately accurate comment that "the majority of those being treated are beyond hope."[14] The provincial government realized the society was not in a position to undertake the construction and operation of a sanatorium for advanced cases. Unwilling to do so itself, the government withdrew the condition attached to its grant on the understanding that advanced cases would continue to be accepted at Tranquille.

Money for the care and treatment of patients presented a separate challenge to the society. During the first three years of operation, these costs averaged $55 to $60 per month per patient, considerably higher than average costs for patient care in other British Columbia hospitals. Aware of public sensitivity about expenditure, society executives regularly explained that the high quality of food, the isolation of Tranquille and the high number of advanced cases inflated the costs considerably. They also made it plain that no patient was denied a bed at Tranquille due to an inability to pay. In fact, few patients paid the facility's full rate of $14 per week. In 1909, for example, only 44 percent of operating revenues came from fee-paying patients, and many of them had fees paid for them by the branch societies. Fagan noted that the operating deficit in 1909 of only $265 would have been much "heavier had not the noble girls of Vancouver and Victoria Auxiliary Societies come to the assistance of patients from their respective cities. Such...are represented as pay patients on the books." The remaining 56 percent of operating revenues came from the regular provincial government's hospital grant and from private subscription.[15] The balance sheet was not helped by the fact that a few of the paying patients neglected to pay their debts upon discharge from the institution.

With nearly 2,000 members and twenty-eight auxiliary societies, the organization Fagan created to provide financial assistance to the society reached its peak in 1910. However, the support of the branch societies went beyond simply providing patient fees. Both Vancouver and Victoria had junior and senior auxiliaries and all four branches were very active. Collectively, they provided sheets and mattresses for the new sanatorium building, as well as a piano, Christmas hampers, and magazines. They also paid for furniture and accessories for the dining room, furniture and equipment in the new building, and the furnishing of several rooms. The contributions of smaller branches were less spectacular, but valuable nevertheless. The Salt Spring Island auxiliary, for example, donated more than fifty dollars raised by a concert and dance. The Kamloops auxiliary became more actively involved in fundraising in 1909 under Marion Hallamore and provided furnishing for a room in the new building. The rooms could not be used until they were furnished, and after the trials of construction, the parent society had no money whatsoever for this purpose.

Appeals to the forty-six municipal governments of the province met with limited success. Nearly half contributed to the building fund in 1908, but many were reluctant to repeat their contributions in the following years. The annual report for 1908 includes the admission that the "financing of the Consumption hospital is a trying proposition."[16] Victoria's mayor Morley grew increasingly irate in 1910 at the society's persistent pursuit of funds. When Fagan requested support for the maintenance of the sanatorium early in the year, Morley demanded a statement of accounts and referred the request to the finance committee. When one of the Victoria women's auxiliaries requested approval for a tag day in October, Morley delivered an extended diatribe on mismanagement at the sanatorium before he granted the request. In December, he demanded a personal and public accounting from a full delegation of the society.

The British Columbia Anti-Tuberculosis Society needed both funds and good fortune if its venture were to succeed and both seemed in short supply. The contract to build the sanatorium had been granted to O'Dell because his had been the low bid. Almost immediately difficulties emerged. Nearly all building material was sent from Vancouver, and the need to unload at Tranquille Siding and barge across the lake caused O'Dell unanticipated delay and expense. The original completion was planned for May 1909, but was soon postponed to the end of June. An inspection in April by a committee of the society revealed that the coastal contractor had not taken into account the realities of winter in the province's Interior and much of the plumbing had been placed outside the building. Further delay resulted while the mistake was corrected. By the middle of the summer, O'Dell advised the society that, though the building was nearly finished, he was financially unable to meet his obligations.

The society had no choice but to take over the completion of the project. Irving later claimed he was appointed "clerk of the works," but, in fact, it was farm superintendent W.W. Shaw to whom the society turned. Many of O'Dell's creditors donated a portion of their materials and Shaw's ranch crew provided the labour when their other duties permitted. Shaw was also able to obtain some additional timber from the Lac du Bois area, just north of the sanatorium. By mid-November, Shaw was able to inform the board that the building was finally complete and ready for furnishing. The board in 1909 had met quarterly and held five emergency meetings to deal with matters of building and equipment. Towards the end of the year, any energy they may have had remaining was taken up by a bitter dispute with their sanatorium superintendent, Dr. Irving.

With the small Tranquille sanatorium filled to capacity, Irving had seen an opportunity to treat patients privately. He attended to the care of tubercular patients at the Cooney ranch and he opened his own private facility in Kamloops, which he attended every Wednesday and Sunday afternoon. He would later argue that the practice was permitted at Gravenhurst and elsewhere, and that the Anti-Tuberculosis Society knew and initially approved of his activities. The board disagreed. Mindful of the strong opposition in Kamloops to the establishment of a sanatorium, the society wanted nothing to provide its opponents with a platform to revive their agitation. In May 1909, the board advised Irving that the constitution of the society specifically required the medical superintendent to "devote his entire time and attention to the welfare of the inmates of the Sanatorium."[17] When Irving ignored the letter, he was summoned to a meeting of the board of directors in Vancouver in October. Neither party was willing to alter its position, and in early January 1910, Irving submitted his resignation to take effect 11 March. The resignation was accepted by the directors with no statement of regret. The dispute received no publicity and Irving quietly announced he would expand his private treatment of tuberculosis in Kamloops. His new fifteen-patient Riverside Cottage Sanatorium, located just outside the city's eastern limits, would cater only to those in incipient stages of the disease and only to those capable of paying the fees. Though the phrase was not in use at the time, a "two-tier system" of tuberculosis treatment had become available in the Kamloops area.

The announcement of Irving's intentions was not well received in Kamloops. Many were concerned that the city was destined to follow the pattern of Gravenhurst where the original sanatorium of 1897 was followed by the establishment of three more institutions within less than a decade. The *Kamloops Standard* assured its readers that Irving's Riverside Cottage Sanatorium was "clean, properly cared for and perfectly sanitary," but the city council sought to limit the numbers of such institutions and to prevent a further influx of tubercular patients. M.S. Wade at the *Inland Sentinel* continued in his familiar vein:

> It is not fair to the poor suffering that, arriving here to find the sanatorium closed to them, the residents mortally afraid of taking them in, the hotels also closed to them, they should be thrown entirely upon their own resources or the tender mercies of more or less charitable strangers.

He concluded that the provincial government should take "a few thousands of the millions they have accumulated" to build a sanatorium for advanced cases.[18] With his conclusion at least, the Anti-Tuberculosis Society had some sympathy. Just a month earlier, at their annual meeting, the Court of Governors passed a resolution formally asking the government to take over the work of the society.

The society's problems continued. As the directors were making plans for a 24 May official opening, they received notification that the forty-acre property at Tranquille claimed by the Chinese settler had been granted to him by the federal government. The society withheld an interest payment due to William Fortune in protest, and placed the matter in the hands of its solicitors, but apparently without success. Due to an inability to furnish the rooms in the new sanatorium, the official opening was again postponed amidst hopes that King Edward would agree to perform the ceremonies. Dr. J.J. Thompson of Esquimalt was appointed to take over as medical superintendent and assumed responsibility on 1 April. Within a short time, he found himself engaged in a dispute with matron Jean Matheson that resulted in his charging her with insubordination and neglect of duty. The board decided to investigate the dispute and eventually expressed its full support of Matheson. However, before the investigation began, Thompson submitted his resignation on 7 July to take effect 25 August. D.W. Davis, a graduate of McGill not yet registered in British Columbia, agreed to supervise the institution (on an interim basis and without pay) while the dismayed board of directors searched for a new medical superintendent.

Ironically, the British Columbia Medical Association made plans to hold its annual convention at Tranquille in the still empty new building in mid-August. The association's new president, Robert Irving of the Riverside Cottage Sanatorium, was responsible for arrangements. One of the scheduled speakers was to be Dr. J.J. Thompson, the outgoing medical superintendent of Tranquille Sanatorium. Perhaps the potential for discord discouraged some from attending. According to one report, only nine doctors were present and that number included Fagan, Irving, and Thompson. Significantly, with Dr. Irving in the chair, the small group unanimously passed a resolution approving of the operation of the Tranquille Sanatorium. Any criticisms or animosities the two former superintendents may have held were not discussed publicly.

While the directors purposely moved slowly in their search for a new medical superintendent "so as to make no mistake this time," they resolved to end the ongoing embarrassment of the unopened new building. Nearly two years had passed since the hopeful sod turning in October 1908. Invitations were sent to all British Columbia's judges, MPs, senators, and mayors, as well as to a wide range of figures in the business community, inviting them to the official opening on 14 September 1910. The public, too, was invited through newspaper notification. This was to be the occasion to justify all the efforts of the past, while motivating society members and the public to greater efforts in the future. The society intended to capitalize fully on it.

A large attendance from Kamloops and a few public officials witnessed the opening by Lieutenant-Governor Thomas Paterson on the late afternoon of 14 September. Several speeches were made. Fagan made a dramatic appeal for sixty-three wealthy British Columbians to donate $1,000 each so the sanatorium could be properly completed. Dr. Procter provided an interesting twist on the founding of the institution by claiming that the "initial movement" to control tuberculosis in British Columbia had come from Kamloops. Kamloops mayor John Robinson spoke, and it was announced with appreciation that Dalton, the architect, had declined to accept his $3,500 fee. All admired the maple hardwood floors and the balconies of the still unfurnished rooms, and after refreshments, visiting dignitaries crossed the lake to catch the late train at Tranquille Siding back to Vancouver. Though successful in itself, the official opening was a failure as an exercise in publicity. Perhaps because it had been so long anticipated, the event generated little coverage by the newspapers of the province.

In early November, Dr. Davis received his provincial certification (and, at last, a salary) as he agreed to continue as interim superintendent. Finally, an announcement was made in mid-November that Charles Harvey Vrooman of Winnipeg had been appointed medical superintendent at Tranquille. The society had acknowledged that a competitive salary was necessary to attract the kind of commitment to the institution that was required. Dr. Vrooman was to be paid $208 per month plus room and board for himself and his family when he assumed his duties, but his salary would rise to $300 just one year later. At the end of a trying year, members of the Anti-Tuberculosis Society believed they could enjoy, at last, some moments free from anxiety and toil.

They were mistaken. Robert Irving chose the moment of Vrooman's appointment to launch a vigorous attack on the society through the newspapers in Vancouver and Victoria. In early December, he made public the dispute that led to his resignation a year earlier, alleging that Fagan had personally authorized his private treatment of patients and claiming the directors had withheld information from him. He stated that the sanatorium lacked even the simplest medical appliances, and that only the ignorance of the patients there prevented them from criticizing the care they received. The timing of this broadside invites speculation. Perhaps Vrooman's salary represented too considerable an advance beyond his own as superintendent, or perhaps lingering animosities could simply not be restrained any longer. Whatever Irving's motivation might have been, within a few days a letter to the same newspapers from Dr. Thompson echoed his complaints. Thompson said his suggestions about patient admissions were dismissed by Fagan in a cavalier fashion. He insisted the financial mismanagement of the institution was proven by the fact that, though the new building held no patients, a Chinese labourer was employed to clean its windows.

The *Kamloops Standard* did not refer to the doctors' critical letters, but the *Inland Sentinel* was delighted to inform its readers about them. Reprinting both letters, Wade reminded the people of Kamloops that his newspaper had always opposed the establishment of the sanatorium and editorialized that four superintendents in one year was in itself proof of "a faulty administration." He urged the government to act upon the recent recommendation of the British Columbia Union of Municipalities by taking "full and sole control" of the institution immediately.[19] Though this was a position long favoured by many in the society, agitation by the *Inland Sentinel* about incompetence and mismanagement was not the kind of evidence in support of the position they could welcome. A clearly tired and discouraged board of directors confirmed that if the provincial government would take over the operation, it would raise no objection. Individual members probably prayed it would happen quickly.

Chapter Notes

1 University of British Columbia (UBC), Records of the British Columbia Anti-Tuberculosis Society, Court of Governors Book, p. 38.
2 First Annual Report of the Directors the Anti-Tuberculosis Society 1908, p. 9.
3 *Kamloops Standard*, 14 March 1908, p. 8.
4 *Vancouver Daily Province*, 6 April 1908, p. 2.
5 British Columbia Archives and Records Service (BCARS), GR 2866, box 1, file 1, Robert Irving, "The Early Days of Tranquille Sanatorium."
6 BCARS, Additional MSS 1916, Records of the British Columbia Anti-Tuberculosis Society, Letter Book 1908, Fagan to Frank Oliver, 11 April 1908 and Fagan to William Templeman, 17 July 1908.
7 *Kamloops Standard*, 12 November 1908, p. 1 and p. 8; and *Inland Sentinel*, 13 November 1908, p. 1, p. 5, p. 7.
8 National Archives of Canada (NAC), MG 28 I 75, Records of the Canadian Tuberculosis Association, volume VI, file 6, "Tuberculosis or the Bacillus 'at Home'," (Victoria, 1908).
9 BCARS, GD 2866, box 1, file 1, Robert Irving, "The Early Days of Tranquille Sanatorium"; Third Annual Report of the British Columbia Anti-Tuberculosis Society 1910, p. 17.
10 UBC, Records of British Columbia Anti-Tuberculosis Society, Minute Book, Irving to Fagan, 15 October 1909.
11 *Victoria Colonist*, 30 April 1908, p. 7.
12 NAC, MG 28 I 75 volume VI, file 6, Records of the Canadian Tuberculosis Association. British Columbia Anti-Tuberculosis Society, "A Summary of the Work Accomplished," pp. 6-7.
13 Third Annual Report of the British Columbia Anti-Tuberculosis Society 1909, pp. 10-11.
14 *Inland Sentinel*, 8 October 1909, p. 8.
15 Third Annual Report of the Anti-Tuberculosis Society 1909, pp. 7 and 23.
16 Second Annual Report of the Directors of the Anti-Tuberculosis Society 1909, p. 7.
17 UBC, Records of the British Columbia Anti-Tuberculosis Society, Court of Governors, By-Laws, Rules and Regulations, Article 25.
18 *Inland Sentinel*, 24 March 1910, p. 2.
19 *Inland Sentinel*, 2 December 1910, p. 2.

The King Edward Sanatorium: Progress and Stability

The institution taken over by Charles Vrooman at the close of 1910 was an institution in disarray. It was chronically under-funded, with the majority of the forty-nine private rooms for patients in its proud new building still unfurnished and therefore unoccupied. The ranks of its critics had recently been swelled by former medical superintendents. Located near a larger community still sharply divided in its attitude towards it, the Tranquille Sanatorium had been unable to achieve stability. Compounding the difficulties was the decision of Jean Matheson to resign as matron effective 31 December.[1]

It may have provided some comfort had the directors known that their difficulties were not unique. The new Queen Alexandra Sanatorium, for example, which opened in London, Ontario in 1910 would go through four medical superintendents and an equal number of matrons in its first two years of operation as relations between its board and senior staff evolved.[2] However, surviving records suggest strongly that the British Columbia Anti-Tuberculosis Society was isolated from the experience of its counterparts in the rest of the country. When the board met Vrooman officially for the first time at the end of December in Victoria, hopes for a reversal of the society's fortunes were evident. But with only a few months' experience at Manitoba's new sanatorium near Ninette, Vrooman was not the man of extensive experience the directors would have preferred. Vrooman himself was well aware, as were the critics and directors of the Anti-Tuberculosis Society, that he would be subject to considerable scrutiny. Undoubtedly, in some quarters at least, rapid judgements would be made concerning his conduct and abilities.

The criticisms of the conduct and abilities of Dr. Fagan made public by Irving and Thompson could not go unchallenged, and the board authorized Fagan to publicize his responses to them. He did so in a lengthy and vigorous letter published in the *Kamloops Standard* on 6 January 1911. He pointed out that Irving had been present at the meeting of the board in February 1909, when the constitution of the society was amended to state that the superintendent was required to "devote his entire time to the welfare of the inmates." Fagan argued Irving could not have been ignorant of his conditions of employment. He detailed his own actions and statements concerning the allegations brought by Dr. Thompson. He noted that, concerning the dispute between Jean Matheson and Thompson, he had not changed his opinion that Matheson deserved the board's expression of its "complete and entire satisfaction with her work."[3] None of the individuals involved—Fagan, Irving, and Thompson—would ever refer publicly to these matters again.

If their critics had been effectively silenced for the moment, members of the British Columbia Anti-Tuberculosis Society saw little else to encourage them. The general malaise was reflected in a poor attendance at the annual general meeting in February 1911. Delegates were disappointed to hear that the Conservative provincial government would not agree to pay for the construction of a separate institution for advanced cases. Nevertheless, though it continued to fall below expectations, the support of the government was evident. A new provincial statute required each municipal government to pay Tranquille $1 per day for each destitute patient from its locality under treatment at the institution. In addition, a new provincial grant of $30,000 towards the building fund was announced. However, the grant would be received only if the institution continued to treat patients in advanced stages of the disease. The board accepted the condition, however reluctantly. Plans were made to convert the old Fortune ranch houses to suit that purpose and to construct a new sleeping pavilion to the east of the Main Building.

In the Main Building, which was intended for incipient cases only, rooms were slowly becoming available for patient use as they were furnished with money raised by the branch societies and by private donations. The first few patients were accommodated in early December 1910. The Kamloops branch society, despite a sharply reduced membership, managed nevertheless to furnish two rooms. Two other rooms were furnished by a group of Kamloops businessmen which included Neil Dalgleish and Archibald Galloway, both of whom held contracts to supply the institution. Other rooms were furnished by corporate donors. By February 1911, twenty-five rooms were in service, but thirty-six others intended for both patients and female staff remained unfurnished. Significant contributions were made by the very active societies of Vancouver and Victoria. In addition to furnishing several rooms, they provided all the linen and bedding for the bedrooms as well as the cutlery and china for the dining room. The senior Victoria society completely furnished the dining room, while the efforts of the unmarried women of the junior branch raised sufficient funds to pay for all the furnishing required by the kitchen. The board expressed its gratitude, noting the material was "of the first order" and would be "a beautiful and lasting monument to the efforts of the good ladies."[4]

Administrative concerns were also addressed. The discontent expressed by the first three medical superintendents were reconsidered after the controversies had received their public airing. The board, following the practice of other institutions, amended its constitution to allow the medical superintendent "to see cases of tuberculosis privately" and to charge fees for that service. From his private Riverside Cottage Sanatorium at Kamloops, Dr. Irving knew he had won a belated victory. The board also announced its intention to place the day-to-day operation of the institution in the hands of board members resident at Tranquille and Kamloops. The new House Committee was to consist of Dr. Vrooman, ranch manager W.W. Shaw, Kamloops mayor John Robinson, local bank manager A.H. Skey, and any other member of the board of directors who happened to be in Kamloops when meetings occurred. The very busy annual meeting concluded with an expression of deep sorrow at the death of its honorary patron Edward VII. It decided to rename the institution the King Edward Memorial Sanatorium in honour of the king's antituberculosis work throughout the British Empire. With the changes in nomenclature, constitution and organization, and medical staff, the British Columbia Anti-Tuberculosis Society (in conversation, often referred to as the Anti-Tubs) hoped that a new era of stability had begun in its operation of the sanatorium at Tranquille.

The year 1912 saw significant changes at Tranquille. The previous year, the board had decided to erect a sleeping pavilion to accommodate twenty-four patients and another building to serve as an administration building and a residence for both nursing and support staff. A room in the administration building was to be set aside and made available at $2 per night for visiting family or friends. Located just to the east of the Main Building, both buildings were completed only slightly behind schedule in July 1912.

The board wanted to avoid a repetition of the situation when the Main Building had been completed, with rooms empty and unused until funds became available to furnish them one at a time. An offer from the Independent Order of Odd Fellows (IOOF) of British Columbia to take on the responsibility of furnishing the Sleeping Pavilion, therefore, was eagerly accepted. At a final cost of approximately $2,500, the rooms were all "splendidly furnished" by the IOOF and a grateful board decided to place a plaque in the Sleeping Pavilion to acknowledge the contribution. The building was ready for occupation when its construction was completed in July. The ceremonial presentation of furnishing and equipment was made by Odd Fellow E.L. Webber of Penticton in February 1913.[5]

The construction of the Canadian Northern Railway along the north shore of Kamloops Lake also brought great change. The company offered $500 an acre for a corridor of fourteen acres well behind the sanatorium building. Though farm manager Shaw insisted the land was worth $1,000 an acre, the board accepted the offer in January 1912. In March, Vrooman suggested the board could take advantage of the presence of construction equipment and expertise to make significant changes to the terrain around the sanatorium. An arrangement was made to fill ravines and level the ground, with the work being completed by May 1912. The construction and levelling helped to reduce the rattlesnake problem on the sanatorium grounds. When the work was done, both Canadian Northern and its sub-contractor, Schact and Company, donated most of their costs to the Anti-Tuberculosis Society.[6]

The arrival of the railway made the institution much less isolated and significant savings in transportation costs were anticipated. Patients and visitors would no longer have to cross the lake from the CPR's Tranquille Siding or travel from the CPR station in Kamloops. The Canadian Northern's Tranquille station was situated just north of the sanatorium and required only a short drive to the institution. In anticipation of the need to transport people and goods, the sanatorium purchased its first automobile—a Ford—in 1913. Transportation costs from Kamloops were eliminated as freight deliveries went directly to Tranquille. Vrooman estimated that the savings to the institution amounted initially to eight cents per patient per day—a significant amount for an institution usually operating from a deficit situation. Unfortunately, without a station master present, theft of supplies deposited at Tranquille station soon became a serious problem. Once the regular train service began in 1915, it became necessary to have nearly all shipments apart from coal deposited at the Canadian Northern station in Kamloops and trucked to Tranquille, eliminating much of the anticipated reduction in transportation costs.

Patterns of Operation

Relations with the nearby community of Kamloops were still a matter of concern for the sanatorium. However, as the patient population at the sanatorium continued to increase, the business community in Kamloops saw expanding opportunities. Consequently, there were no fresh outbursts of opposition reminiscent of the Anti-Sanitarium (in Kamloops) League. Surviving fragmentary business records suggest that, amongst others, the Dalgleish firm of Kamloops, the Hudson's Bay Company, and the Charles Cooney ranch adjacent to the sanatorium enjoyed significant commerce with the institution.[7] As the fears of contagion diminished, residents of the city also took advantage of employment opportunities at the Alexandra Ranch and at the sanatorium itself. Ranch work was available, mostly on a seasonal basis, while full-time employment was available for kitchen workers and orderlies. Exclusive of the superintendent, matron, and the ranch staff, the monthly payroll was nearly $700 by early 1911.[8]

Financial considerations notwithstanding, the society had learned from experience that fear of contagion in Kamloops could easily find expression in hostility towards the institution. In February 1911, when the city's medical health officer raised a concern about unsanitary conditions, Mayor John Robinson declared emphatically that the owners of local hotels and boarding houses should be prosecuted if any of their tenants were found to be tubercular. Council then passed a resolution requiring police to enforce the city's anti-spitting by-law. Clearly, concerns that the institution and Irving's private clinic were drawing an unhealthy population to the area were very much alive.

Perhaps to address these concerns, within a year of Dr. Vrooman's arrival at Tranquille, the board began to release the superintendent's monthly reports to the local newspapers. The reports indicated the number of patients admitted and discharged, and acknowledged contributions of goods and services from branch societies, residents, and businesses. The monthly reports did not disguise the realities of the disease being treated. Financial details, waiting lists, and deaths were also mentioned regularly. Additional publicity for the cause was generated by the activities of the Kamloops branch society, rejuvenated after 1912 under the leadership of Susan Wood. Tag days and social events were held to raise funds for the maintenance account at the sanatorium and to provide care for poorer victims of tuberculosis from Kamloops, whether they were at the sanatorium or not. Mrs. Wood declared that the women of Kamloops were "every bit as interested in public matters as the men," adding that, when it came to antituberculosis work, the women were distinctly more interested than the men.

People involved in the work of the society had become well aware of the requirements of public education. An official pamphlet was produced in 1912 to make people aware of the nature of the programme of treatment followed at the sanatorium. Intended primarily for prospective patients, it also served to inform the public of policies and procedures, and to promote the healthful atmosphere of the institution. A photograph of fruit-laden branches is included. Another photograph, over the caption "Tubercular Terrors Lost in Mirthful Pastime," shows ambulant patients skating on Kamloops Lake. In conversation with visitors, Dr. Vrooman was fond of saying that the greatest curative agents in the fight against tuberculosis were "sunshine, fresh air and a stout heart." To this list, he would quickly add "rest, good food and graduated exercise."

An extensive report in the *Kamloops Standard* in July 1914 contributed to the information campaign. It provided a description of the general routine followed at Tranquille:

> Those who imagine that the sanatorium at Tranquille is a sort of convalescent hostelry where patients come and rest and bask in the sun, get up at whatever time they please and generally live the free and easy life of the modern health resort will be surprised at the real condition which a visit to the sanatorium will reveal. Running through the entire routine at Tranquille is a firm, albeit kindly, discipline. Perhaps...a patient will be somewhat startled when he is told by the medical superintendent to stay in bed for a week or perhaps a month or more after his arrival. When the time comes for him to be allowed to get up his exercise is graduated for him on a carefully arranged basis.
>
> This is the first great factor in the treatment: — Rest.
>
> On the day following his admission to the sanatorium, the medical superintendent makes a thorough physical examination of the patient. He is thoroughly sounded and the extent of the disease is diagnosed by the physician. This examination is recorded on a large chart, part of which shows an anatomical reproduction of the human frame on which is carefully traced the extent of the cavities or diseased areas.
>
> From this time forward the patient becomes a study to the medical superintendent and his staff of nurses. Twice daily his pulse, temperature and respiration are recorded on a chart. When he shows signs of improvement he is gradually advanced to the stage of light exercise, which is slowly increased as improvement is shown.[9]

The goal of treatment was to achieve the physical restoration of the patient, while encouraging the habits and self-discipline that would be required after the patient left the institution. Patients were expected to follow the prescribed daily routine of the sanatorium. Breakfast was served at 8 a.m., followed by rest on the verandahs, graduated exercise for some, other meals as the day progressed, and more rest before "lights out" at 9:30 p.m. Conversation about the disease was discouraged. Alcohol was strictly forbidden and immediate discharge from the institution was threatened if the prohibition were broken. Seen from a late twentieth-century perspective, the management of the sanatorium was curiously tolerant of tobacco, allowing patients to smoke on the verandahs and outside the buildings. Surgical intervention was also added to the methods of treatment. Artificial pneumothorax, which is an induced collapse of an affected lung allowing it to rest, was made available to selected Tranquille patients after December 1913.

No one who had been resident of British Columbia for at least six months was refused entry, even if there was an inability to pay the institution's fees. The average cost of treatment for each patient was approximately $2 per day during the pre-war years. The society optimistically had hoped to charge $25 per week for rooms in the new Main Building, but quickly found this impractical. Many wealthier victims of the disease chose treatment at home or in private sanatoria, whereas poorer victims required the financial assistance of the provincial and municipal governments.

The proportion of less affluent and indigent patients rose steadily. Only thirty-eight of the 218 patients treated in 1913 paid the full rate of $15 per week. Nearly seventy patients were able to pay only partial rates; fifty-seven had their fees paid for by their municipalities, and fifty-three more had no support whatsoever. After collecting more than $15,000 from patients and after receiving payments from municipalities and the province of more than $35,000, the deficit in the maintenance account still amounted to $15,000 in 1913. This was nearly triple the deficit of the previous year and represented a figure that frustrated even the best efforts of the branch societies.[10] After the first few years of enthusiasm, the number of active branch societies shrank to half a dozen, with only the four societies of Vancouver and Victoria contributing substantially. Fundraising efforts were further frustrated by the sharp economic depression that had taken hold of the province. Dr. Fagan's hopes of steady income from the charitable work of women's auxiliaries had initially been satisfied, but by 1912 he was forced to admit that "such assistance has not been forthcoming."[11]

Attempts were made to reduce costs by reducing service to poorer patients. The board considered (but did not adopt) a proposal by Director W.F. Wood of Kamloops to accommodate non-paying patients in tents and cottages and to provide them with a lower quality of food. However, the informational pamphlet issued by the sanatorium makes it quite clear that a reduced level of service was provided to the poor. It states that patients who were not paying the full rates were "required to make their own beds and keep their lockers in good order." They were also "expected to perform any other work assigned to them by the physician...without detriment to their health."[12] In other words, poorer patients provided a certain amount of unpaid labour. The society was struggling with the contradiction between operating an institution largely for the poor and the needs of financial self-sufficiency. The Sleeping Pavilion, intended for twenty-four patients, was soon accommodating thirty-two.

The board was dismayed by the size of the 1913 deficit. Convinced that the geographic distance between Victoria and Tranquille increased administrative costs, the board resolved to move "the active management of the Society and the Sanatorium" to Kamloops in 1914. At its annual general meeting in March 1914, the board refused to proceed until the government gave some indication that it was aware of the seriousness of the situation. Without increased assistance, it threatened to "clear up the Society's responsibilities, close the Sanatorium, and dispose of the Society's affairs according to its constitution."[13] Sympathetic and supportive as ever, the government nevertheless was unwilling to assume responsibility for the institution and unable to increase its financial support due to its own increasing economic difficulties. Therefore, the government took the unusual step of allowing part of its building grant to Tranquille to be used to offset the deficit and promised to require an increase in municipal support to $1.25 per day per patient in 1915. Board member and cattle baron Pat Burns helped the situation by promising an annual donation of $2,000 as long as the sanatorium remained open. Though the deficit was thereby reduced to just over $5,500 in 1914, the threat of closure was repeated at the annual meeting in February 1915. The society received strong editorial support from newspapers in Vancouver, and the agitation resulted in a donation of $7,000 from Vancouver City Council.[14] Nevertheless, the constant concern about finances would continue to be the chief discouragement to those who felt the institution should continue to be privately operated.

Another source of discouragement to the Anti-Tuberculosis Society was the increasing number of patients who entered the institution in an advanced stage. Many of the poorer patients had remained at work during the incipient stage of the disease, entering the sanatorium only when debilitated, with a sharply diminished chance of being cured. Desirous of treating such patients and required by conditions of their government funding to do so, the board nevertheless stated repeatedly that a separate facility was required for them. Repeatedly, the board pointed out that the sanatorium had been established to combat the disease in its incipient stages, not to provide long-term care for those who had little hope of a cure.

The society's annual reports note with dismay that the majority of those being admitted were in advanced stages of the disease and that this prevented the admission of patients whose chances of being cured were much greater. More than forty people were on the waiting list in 1913 and Vrooman pointed out that the transportation of advanced cases to Tranquille from the lower mainland was in addition both futile and expensive. Sixty percent of admissions in 1913 were described as "far advanced." The attempt to segregate the two classes of patients was short-lived. The larger of the two old ranch buildings that had served as the original sanatorium buildings was being used to house the advanced cases but was deteriorating rapidly. In 1913, the board formally proposed again that the government should provide $100,000 for the construction of a separate modern building for advanced cases.[15] The proposal was turned down. The board then declared the old ranch houses were unsuitable for treatment of any kind, and abandoned them in November 1913. Both incipient and advanced cases were thereafter accommodated in the Main Building—a combination that Fagan had noted, as early as 1902, would be highly discouraging to patients in the early stage of the disease. Men and women were accommodated on separate floors.

Though it is difficult to attempt a picture of the "average patient" at the sanatorium, it is possible nevertheless to identify some general characteristics. The patient population at the institution was predominantly male, with women patients being outnumbered by a ratio of as much as three to one. In the immediate pre-war years, however, the number of women patients increased steadily and by 1914, women made up more than a third of the patients. Socially, the patients were drawn largely from the working population of the province. Wealthier victims generally avoided confinement in the sanatorium by paying for private care.

Patients, typically, were between the ages of fifteen and forty-five. Few children were admitted, though their numbers were beginning to increase. By 1914, Dr. Vrooman was becoming anxious to create a separate children's ward and to see to it that schooling was offered. An adult patient conducted an open-air school for nine young patients, but instruction for the children was dependent upon there being a willing and capable adult amongst the patient population. The Kamloops branch society paid for the construction of a separate children's balcony in 1915, and a brass plaque acknowledging the contribution was placed in the front balcony of the Main Building.[16]

Racially, the population was overwhelmingly of European descent. Very rarely, a non-white patient would be accepted, but the occasions were so few they only proved the rule that medical treatment in British Columbia early in the century was the preserve of the white population. Though much higher rates of infection were found among the Chinese and Native inhabitants of the province, their admittance to the sanatorium was seldom even contemplated by either the victims themselves or their medical attendants. The separate Chinese hospital in Vancouver had fully half its available beds taken by Chinese tuberculosis patients. Natives, on the other hand, were not treated at all. As wards of the federal government, they were not considered a provincial responsibility. However, the federal government had no treatment programme or facility available for them. The typical patient at the King Edward Sanatorium at Tranquille, therefore, was a male of European descent, youthful or in early middle age, unable to pay the weekly fees, and suffering from an advanced stage of the disease.

The medical staff consisted of Dr. Vrooman, an assistant medical superintendent after 1912, the matron, and, once the capacity of eighty-eight patients was reached with the opening of the Sleeping Pavilion, perhaps as many as seven nurses. Having agreed to pay a significant salary to Dr. Vrooman, the board was hard pressed to offer competitive wages to the rest of its staff. In fact, the first assistant superintendent initially received no salary at all. Financial constraints and the relative isolation of the institution may explain the difficulty the board had in attracting a matron who was committed to long-term employment. Unsatisfactory accommodation was also a factor until the new dual-purpose Nurses' Home and Administration Building was opened in July 1912. After the departure of Jean Matheson in December 1910, two successive matrons stayed in the job for only one year each. However, with the appointment of Mary Thomas in early 1913 at a salary of $60 per month, the institution again had a matron prepared to stay for a longer term.

Surviving records of the British Columbia Anti-Tuberculosis Society make few references to the regular nursing staff. Names are mentioned rarely and terms of service are not noted. Even the number of nurses employed given above is speculative. Similarly, there is little information about the non-medical staff. Cooks, kitchen help and female orderlies were the occupations available, but practically no information about numbers employed and salaries paid is included in the society's annual reports. Accommodation at Tranquille, especially for married employees, was scarce. The Main Building had room for only sixteen nurses or maids. However, until the war years, complaints of a rapid staff turnover do not appear in the annual reports. What does occur is an indication of the perils of providing care for tubercular patients: two of the institution's nurses developed pulmonary tuberculosis in 1913.[17]

Information about the Alexandra Ranch, during the early years, is also fragmentary. The stock at the end of 1907 was comprised of 600 cattle, 200 chickens, 65 horses, 18 sheep, and 12 pigs. The intention of converting the ranch quickly to dairy and poultry was thwarted by financial constraints and other priorities at the sanatorium. To keep pace with egg consumption, the number of chickens increased to 600 by the end of 1908. A boarding house for twenty men, a new barn, and a slaughterhouse were constructed. Except for the two ranch houses, the dilapidated Fortune buildings were demolished in 1909. A residence was constructed for W.W. Shaw in 1909, and the beginning of a dairy herd was acquired. Shaw was soon able to report that all dairy cattle were "tuberculin tested and found free of disease."

By the end of 1909, Shaw was also able to report that "the buildings on the Ranch now are almost sufficient to meet the requirements of the Sanatorium."

Unlike the sanatorium itself, the ranch was a profitable operation. Money was raised through the sale of excess stock. Although occasional outside purchases were required, the production of fruits and vegetables, eggs, meats, and milk were generally sufficient for the needs of the sanatorium. Ranch profits provided much-needed funds for the sanatorium, or, more frequently, paid for repairs and improvements required by the ranch itself. At a board meeting held in Kamloops in March 1913, Shaw recommended that the ranch operation shift further into dairying, with most horses and beef cattle being put up for sale. The board agreed, and prepared to seek government assistance for the acquisition of thoroughbred stock. Shaw would not oversee the implementation of the developments he recommended. At the same board meeting, he announced his intention to retire.

His successor, David Strachan, began his duties in April 1914. He was a dairyman and was pleased to oversee the development of the dairy herd. In June, he was authorized to send several of the Alexandra Ranch's beef cattle to the Colony Farm at New Westminster in exchange for eight pedigreed dairy cows and a bull. The sheep and pig stocks were also improved. In 1915, he planted the first alfalfa crop at the ranch with such success that the acreage under alfalfa was steadily expanded, and, in good years, would later provide three or even four crops annually. One Vancouver newspaper credited Strachan with having "turned the Alexandra Ranch into a show place."[18] Every year, Strachan was proud to be able to report to the board on awards for fruits and vegetables and prizes for livestock received at both the Kamloops and Vancouver exhibitions.

Though the presence of Tranquille Creek had been one of the factors inducing the board to purchase the Fortune property in 1907, problems of water supply required attention. The creek was useful for irrigation purposes, but could not be used for drinking water because horses and cattle fouled its contents. Wells were, therefore, required. To supply the increased number of patients after the new building opened, Shaw constructed a six thousand-gallon tank atop a fifty-foot tower in 1909. Completed at a cost of over $2,000, the tower was fed by a good spring-fed well, with a small gas-powered pump providing water to the tower. Though the quality of the water was good, the system could not supply an adequate amount of water for drinking and for the fire protection at the same time. An additional well was needed by 1913, and another in 1917. Not until mid-1918 did Vrooman express some satisfaction with the water supply.

Water for irrigation purposes was drawn from behind a dam that was built about a mile from the mouth of Tranquille Creek. There was an ample supply of water in spring and early summer, but it was inadequate in late summer and fall. Strachan suggested the construction of a dam at the headwaters of Tranquille Lake, some thirty miles from the sanatorium, to create a reservoir for late season use. With the cooperation of the Cooney family and their agreement to pay half the $900 cost of construction, Strachan and his Alexandra Ranch staff built the dam in the late summer of 1918. The dam was a success, but was washed away in the spring. A stronger and more durable dam was constructed in 1919. The Strachan dam was able to provide the combined Cooney and Alexandra ranches with all their irrigation requirements for many years.

The sewage system, too, required attention and repair as early as 1908 when leakage was discovered. A surprise visit from Frank De Grey, Provincial Hospital Inspector, in May 1915 resulted in a report highly complimentary to the institution in all aspects except concerning sewage treatment. De Grey reported that the septic disposal of sewage from the institution was accomplished with "flagrant inefficiency." He added that it was "a most serious menace to the Institution and to the Public Health, and must be attended to without delay. The present condition is little short of criminal."[19] Due to financial constraints, the "menace to the Institution" remained for more than a year until the contract for a new septic tank was finally awarded to the Kamloops firm of Johnston and Company in July 1916. If staff and able patients were permitted to swim in Kamloops Lake before De Grey's visit, they were certainly forbidden to do so afterwards.

It was perhaps the growing number of children at Tranquille who felt this prohibition most strongly. In the spring of 1914, the

Tranquille School opened to serve the families of local ranchers and employees of the King Edward Sanatorium. Twelve students initially attended the school, whose first trustees were Dr. Vrooman, Edmund Cooney, and C. Fredericks. The first teacher, Emily Carey, boarded at the Cooney ranch. David Strachan was the auditor. With 46 recorded visits by trustees and 113 visits by other adults, the Tranquille School was probably the most "visited" school in the province in 1915.[20] The community at Tranquille was also large enough by May 1916 to allow the establishment of a separate post office.

The end of an era for the institution was marked in 1914 by the deaths of two men who had played important roles in establishing the sanatorium at Tranquille. William Fortune, in failing health, sought to conclude his affairs and, as a result, finally agreed to acknowledge that the Anti-Tuberculosis Society should be compensated for the forty acres granted to the Chinese settler. The board readily accepted his offer to reduce the mortgage by $600 and Fortune signed the conveyance papers just before he died in late November 1914. The remaining $20,000 due the Fortune estate was payable in November 1919 and interest at six percent was payable half yearly.[21]

Dr. Fagan did not survive to learn of this settlement. Officially, he continued as secretary to the British Columbia Anti-Tuberculosis Society until 1912 and remained on the executive of the Canadian Association for the Prevention of Tuberculosis. However, declining health had required him to withdraw from an active role in the affairs of both organizations. His death in February 1914 saddened the British Columbia Anti-Tuberculosis Society, which recognized that it had lost its leader and mentor. In a tribute to him, the board in its *Eighth Report* stated: "The Sanatorium at Tranquille and the cause generally throughout the Province will remain a lasting monument to his memory."

Chapter Notes

1 Jean Matheson left Tranquille to become matron at the Royal Inland Hospital in Kamloops, and volunteered for overseas duties during World War I. She was decorated by George V for her services at Salonika. Upon her return to Canada, Matheson began a long tenure as matron at Shaughnessy Military Hospital in Vancouver. When she died in 1938, memorial services were held in both Vancouver and Winnipeg. Her obituary in the Kamloops newspaper contains no mention of her time at the Tranquille Sanatorium. See *Kamloops Sentinel*, 29 April 1938, p. 5.

2 J.T.H. Connor, *A Heritage of Healing*, (London, Ontario: 1990) p. 33.

3 *Kamloops Standard*, 6 January 1911, p. 2.

4 University of British Columbia (UBC), Records of the British Columbia Anti-Tuberculosis Society, Court of Governors, Report of the Board of Governors, 10 February 1911.

5 *Inland Sentinel*, 17 February 1913, p. 1.

6 UBC, Records of the British Columbia Anti-Tuberculosis Society, Minute Book, Report to the Board by Dr. Fagan, 31 May 1912.

7 Kamloops Museum Archives (KMA), Charles T. Cooney Papers, file 69.5.2; British Columbia Archives and Records Service (BCARS), GR 2654, box 1, file 1.

8 UBC, Records of the British Columbia Anti-Tuberculosis Society, Minute Book, 10 February 1911.

9 *Kamloops Standard*, 7 July 1914, p. 4.

10 *Seventh Annual Report of the British Columbia Anti-Tuberculosis Society*, p. 48.

11 UBC, Records of the British Columbia Anti-Tuberculosis Society, Minute Book, Report to the Board by Dr. Fagan, 31 May 1912.

12 BCARS, King Edward Memorial Sanatorium pamphlet (Victoria, 1912).

13 UBC, Records of the British Columbia Anti-Tuberculosis Society, Court of Governors, Minutes of the Seventh Annual General Meeting, 18 March 1914.

14 See 25 February 1915 editions of the *Vancouver News-Advertiser*, *Vancouver Province, and Vancouver Sun.*

15 *Seventh Annual Report of the British Columbia Anti-Tuberculosis Society*, p. 7.

16 *Ninth Annual Report of the British Columbia Anti-Tuberculosis Society*, p. 24.

17 *Seventh Annual Report of the British Columbia Anti-Tuberculosis Society*, p. 28.

18 *Vancouver Province*, 5 June 1916.

19 UBC, Records of the British Columbia Anti-Tuberculosis Society, Minute Book, Board Meeting 23 June 1915.

20 British Columbia *Sessional Papers* 1916, Forty-Fourth Annual Report of the Public Schools of British Columbia, p. Alxxxvi.

21 UBC, Records of the British Columbia Anti-Tuberculosis Society, Minute Book, Board Meetings of 19 June 1914, 30 December 1914, and 24 February 1915. (Curiously, the society's *Tenth Report* states that no compensation was received for "the Chinaman's ranch.")

The King Edward Sanatorium: Soldiers and Politics

During the fine summer of 1914, the outbreak of war in Europe must have seemed distant and almost illusory from the perspective of the King Edward Sanatorium. Anticipating, like the rest of the country, a successful conclusion to a brief conflict, the staff, patients and board of the British Columbia Anti-Tuberculosis Society did not imagine that the institution could be much affected. In this, they were profoundly mistaken. The war years would see the disruption of funding patterns, difficulties in staffing, the involvement of the federal government in the institution's affairs, and an alteration in the make-up of the patient population.

Administration and Finance

With the great majority of its supporters concentrated in the lower mainland and Victoria, the attempt to transfer the society's "active management" to Kamloops proved impractical. However, even before the death of Fagan, the centre of the society's affairs shifted distinctly from Victoria to Vancouver. Annual meetings of the Court of Governors were held in Vancouver from 1913 onwards, and, increasingly, executive positions on the board of directors were taken by residents of the lower mainland. After the early war years, the society operated from the Board of Trade building in Vancouver. No longer would the medical superintendent of the sanatorium have to include crossing the Strait of Georgia in his travel plans.

It did not take long for the requirements of a nation at war to affect the fundraising abilities of the Anti-Tuberculosis Society. The society had noted the decline in donations by branch societies in the immediate pre-war years, and quickly realized that appeals to a public already supporting war causes would have little positive effect. The four core communities of Kamloops, Vancouver, Victoria, and New Westminster continued to support branch societies' appeals on behalf of the institution, but contributions from these sources would never again match those of 1909-10. Only the Kamloops and New Westminster branch societies would emerge at the end of the war as auxiliaries operating as originally envisioned by Dr. Fagan.

The junior and senior branches in Victoria merged in 1915 and, led by Elinor Hannington, soon amalgamated with the Victorian Order of Nurses, an organization with a mandate much broader than the single cause of antituberculosis work. In 1917 the Vancouver society, led by Catherine Harrison, persuaded the city to assume responsibility for its work, arguing that the task was too great for a private organization. Logically, the city council focussed on local concerns and pursued treatment in Vancouver as a goal. The Rotary Club of Vancouver had begun to take an active interest in tuberculosis treatment, and, by 1916, was caring for fifteen families on a home-care basis. The members of the Vancouver branch society followed the example of the Victoria women and decided to continue their charitable work with the Victorian Order of Nurses. Though the Vancouver branch did not officially disband, it was apparent that the King Edward Sanatorium would be receiving little further benefit from the charitable efforts of dedicated branch societies in Vancouver and Victoria.

The New Westminster branch, led by Mrs. J. Gauvreau, continued to pay fees at Tranquille for poor New Westminster patients. However, by 1917, it was urging the federal government to take over responsibility for treatment of tuberculosis nationwide—an argument Dr. Fagan had personally made to Prime Minister Laurier in 1904. Though their efforts on behalf of Tranquille remained strong, the members of the New Westminster auxiliary devoted some of their energies to the new ward for advanced tuberculosis cases that opened at the Royal Columbian Hospital in 1916. With Susan Wood and Isabel Costley as long-serving executive members, the smaller Kamloops society, formed almost reluctantly in 1907, was becoming the most significant branch society in the province.

Ironically, the year 1915 saw the society able to boast for the first time that it had become self-supporting. The provincial government requirement that municipalities raise their contributions to $1.25 per day per patient certainly helped the accounts at Tranquille, and the board more aggressively pursued those municipalities who demurred. Enderby, for example, saw court proceedings launched for non-payment in 1915. Diminished contributions from branch societies were more than offset by large private donations. Pat Burns continued to make annual contributions of $2,000, and the Free Masons began annual donations of $500 in 1915. Through private donations, provincial government support, and, eventually, contributions from the federal government for the growing number of soldiers after 1915, the operating account managed to stay in the black almost until towards the end of the war.

During the early years of the sanatorium's operation, Dr. Fagan had often appealed to the wealthy few of British Columbia to make significant contributions. In 1915, the board was pleased to learn at last that the appeal had not been ignored. In his will, Joseph Greaves, part owner of the Douglas Lake Ranch, forty miles south of Kamloops, left a significant portion of his wealth to charity. He reversed his initial intention to benefit the Provincial Old Men's Home and the Royal Inland Hospital, both of which were in Kamloops. At the time of his death, it was announced that the two main beneficiaries were to be the Royal Columbian Hospital in New Westminster and the British Columbia Anti-Tuberculosis Society. The will stipulated that one-third of the estate was to be used by the society "only for Anti-Tuberculosis purposes." The board was even more pleased when it eventually learned that the Greaves estate was much larger than anticipated and would provide a bequest to the society of approximately $100,000.[1]

The year 1915 brought more good news for the society when the Conservative provincial government, increasingly worried about its declining political fortunes, promised $75,000 for the construction of a facility to treat advanced cases. The prospect of adequate separate facilities for the treatment of both incipient and advanced cases finally seemed within reach. Plans were made and tenders were called for the new building. A sense of renewed optimism returned to the British Columbia Anti-Tuberculosis Society for the first time in many years.

Casualties of War and Tuberculosis

At Tranquille, the long war in Europe began to affect the make-up of the patient population by the end of 1915. The Canadian Expeditionary Force was involved in actions along the Western Front, and initially its casualties were treated in England. Pressure of numbers in hospital facilities there soon required that convalescent Canadian soldiers be returned to Canada. The federal government, recognizing that treatment of war casualties would require long-term and systematic programmes, set up the Military Hospitals Commission (MHC) in June 1915. Headed by the Conservative Senate leader James Lougheed, the mandate of the commission was to ensure that returned soldiers were provided with appropriate medical care in their province of residence. As numbers of returned convalescent soldiers continued to escalate, the responsibilities of the MHC expanded quickly. By the end of 1916, twenty-eight institutions were being operated by the MHC and facilities at fifteen others were being used. One of them was the King Edward Sanatorium at Tranquille.[2]

It quickly became apparent that the most serious problem facing the Military Hospitals Commission was the care of tubercular soldiers. With Tranquille filled to capacity and with the tuberculosis wards at Vancouver General Hospital and Royal Columbian Hospital also filled, there were no facilities in British Columbia capable of meeting military requirements. On a visit to British Columbia on MHC business, Senator Lougheed held discussions with members of the board of the Anti-Tuberculosis Society. He was told that arrangements could be made at the King Edward Sanatorium if the MHC would pay for the construction of "some temporary additional buildings."[3] Further discussions resulted in a commitment by the Military Hospitals Commission to bear part of the cost of a new sleeping pavilion. The provincial government was to expend $10,000, while the MHC agreed to donate $2,500 towards the construction of the new building. The involvement of the federal government in tuberculosis care, so long desired by the society in peacetime, had occurred as a result of wartime realities. By the summer of 1916, the board formally agreed to set aside as many as thirty-two beds at Tranquille for tubercular military patients, primarily from British Columbia. The Military Hospitals Commission agreed to pay the society $10 per week for each military patient.[4] Located just to the west of the Main Building, the new pavilion opened in the fall of 1916 with accommodation for twenty-two patients. For the first time, serious attention was given to landscaping at the institution, as a number of trees and shrubs were donated by the chairman of the board of directors, Edward Mahon.

The first two soldier patients arrived at Tranquille towards the end of 1915. Their numbers increased steadily, and during 1916 forty-six soldier-patients received treatment at the facility. The continuing war placed increasing pressure on Canada's hospital facilities and, by the end of the year, the number of military patients at Tranquille began to rise sharply. It was anticipated that the thirty-two beds available would soon prove inadequate. Complaints were beginning to be heard that the arrangement for military patients at Tranquille meant denying care to civilian patients. An increase in the number of beds reserved for soldier patients was not an option. The MHC, therefore, decided to refurbish the abandoned Canadian Pacific hotel at Balfour in West Kootenay and to operate it as a military sanatorium. The Balfour Sanatorium opened in April 1917 with a capacity to treat seventy patients.

Across the country, it was not long before discipline problems arose with hospitalized soldiers, and these problems were particularly acute in the tuberculosis hospitals. The soldiers apparently felt more keenly the combination of enforced inactivity and strict behaviour requirements than did the civilian patients. Some insisted they could take orders only from a superior officer and not from civilian doctors. Many refused to do tasks that were required of all able-bodied patients—the most significant of these tasks being the cleaning of lavatories. The King Edward Sanatorium and the other tuberculosis hospitals all faced the same difficulties with the issues of discipline in soldier-patients. Soldier-patients at the Queen Alexandra Sanatorium in London, Ontario petitioned the Military Hospitals Commission for the removal of the medical superintendent there. By the summer of 1916, the Muskoka Free Hospital for Consumptives at Gravenhurst was pressing the MHC for significant changes in regulations and the Laurentian Sanatorium returned fifteen percent of its military patients to their units for disciplinary reasons. Because of the widespread unrest, an order-in-council created the Military

Hospitals Command to deal with matters of discipline and the discharge of military personnel from hospitals.[5]

In May 1916, Dr. Vrooman expelled three soldier-patients from the sanatorium for having gone to Kamloops without permission, probably to enjoy a drink at a local hotel. The three responded to their expulsion by submitting their version of the events that led to their discharge, along with complaints from several other soldier-patients. They included in their submission that most damning of World War I accusations, stating that Dr. Vrooman was pro-German. Vrooman explained to the board that he made no distinctions between military and civilian patients, and that the returned soldiers frequently refused to do the work that was expected of all patients who were able. When further complaints were received later in the summer, the provincial authorities decided to investigate.

The Provincial Board of Health, rather ironically, asked former superintendent Robert Irving to investigate conditions at Tranquille single-handedly. Irving's report bears no trace of the bitterness towards the institution that he held six years earlier. Though he commented on the discomfort caused to patients by the mosquito population, he stated clearly that allegations of poor food, mistreatment and unsatisfactory conditions were "without foundation." He recommended that a military officer be placed in command of soldier patients and that a home visit, prior to admission, should occur to judge whether the prospective soldier-patient would be a satisfactory resident at the institution. He also urged that non-paying patients (that is, the poor and the military) be segregated from paying patients. Action would be taken only on the first of these recommendations.[6]

The difficulties at Tranquille and elsewhere raised the possibility that institutions might refuse to accept additional military patients just as the need for placements was beginning to escalate significantly. The Military Hospitals Commission, therefore, acted quickly and decisively in the summer of 1916 by issuing regulations that made all soldier-patients a casualty command—a unit of both the Canadian Army and the Military Hospitals Command. Doctors' orders about work, rest, and exercise were thereby given the force of military orders, which soldier-patients were not at liberty to refuse.

Insubordinate soldiers could no longer be expelled from hospitals solely by medical superintendents, but would face all the rigours of military discipline instead. Though soldiers did not immediately become model patients as a result, the number of disputes with civilian doctors and medical superintendents declined sharply at Tranquille and nationwide.

Against this background, the operation of the sanatorium with all its challenges and difficulties continued. The annual reports issued by the society regularly lamented that the numbers of advanced cases being treated prevented the institution from carrying out its intended mandate—the treatment of incipient tuberculosis. When a German-speaking woman arrived as a patient, Dr. Vrooman urged the board to require her to enter a private institution. He noted that many English-speaking women were on the waiting list and that many soldier-patients would be upset at her presence. The board supported Vrooman's recommendation. The Vancouver contractor who had built the new sleeping pavilion was asked for restitution when a windstorm blew off part of the roof and caused damage to screens and windows. Dental treatment was begun in January 1917. No Kamloops dentist would agree to take the contract, so a Vancouver dentist spent six days at the sanatorium and agreed to return two or three times a year.

Matron Mary Thomas joined the Queen Alexandra Imperial Nursing Service and went overseas in the spring of 1917. It was at this time that the inflationary pressures of the war became apparent. Her replacement, Mary Ferguson, was appointed at a salary of $65 per month. The wages of first-year nurses were raised to $45 per month on the recommendation of Vrooman, who was becoming concerned about the institution's ability to retain staff. Just over a year later, the wages of first-year nurses rose to $55 a month. Vrooman's own salary had been increased to $3,900 annually in January, while ranch manager Strachan saw his salary raised to $1,800 in August. (Both Strachan and Vrooman enjoyed rent-free accommodation with free heat and light.) Costs of supplies and materials also increased. The small operating surplus recorded in 1917 would be the last.

Provincial politics unavoidably played a role in the deliberations of the society. During the early war years, three directors sat on the board as appointees of the provincial government, but nothing in the surviving records suggests their views differed from those of the rest of the board. Nevertheless, the society was increasingly dependent upon the government due to its own diminished capital and its lessened ability to raise funds. By 1917, operating grants, capital expenditure and amounts paid by municipalities were all determined by Victoria. Essentially, all the society could do was supplement government revenues with its own limited resources.

Soon after the election of the new Liberal administration in November 1916, the society took the opportunity to inform the incoming government of its work and to explain its difficulties. The focus of the submission was the familiar issue of being required to treat advanced cases, contrary to the society's original mandate and intentions. Pointing out that tuberculosis rates were rising in the province's cities, the board asked for a commitment of $150,000 to build new facilities to treat all incipient cases at Tranquille. It recommended the treatment of advanced cases elsewhere, preferably in separate tuberculosis wards in other hospitals. Failing such a commitment, the letter concluded by asking the government to take over the society's work. It was the third time in a decade that the request had been formally made. The board was encouraged by the government's reply that it would "deal in a serious and broad manner" with the issue at the next session of the legislature.[7]

The promise was not kept, but indications of the government's intentions were sufficient to prevent a repetition of the call for a government takeover at the annual general meeting held in February 1918. Though the proposal concerning the treatment of advanced cases at other hospitals would not be acted upon, Provincial Secretary John McLean publicly declared his support for the idea. The government modestly increased its contribution to the operation of the sanatorium and indicated its willingness to share with the federal government the financing of a large new building at Tranquille for soldiers. To acknowledge the extent of its dependence upon public funds, the society altered its by-laws early in 1918 to increase the number of provincially-appointed directors to four. It also permitted two directors to be appointed by the British Columbia Union of Municipalities. Though not a majority on the sixteen-member board, the appointed representatives clearly could carry an influence greater than their numbers warranted. Somewhat ironically, the provincial government chose as its fourth appointee the strongest critic the society had ever faced in its early days. His previous views notwithstanding, former *Inland Sentinel* editor M.S. Wade was appointed to both the board and the House Committee in Kamloops in 1918.

Apart from questions of finance, matters related to the war and the treatment of military patients continued to dominate the affairs of the institution. The community at Tranquille received wide attention by subscribing $15,000 to the last Victory Loan of 1917, $3,350 coming from the soldier-patients.[8] A visit from Governor General the Duke of Devonshire provided encouragement all round. Patriotism notwithstanding, another round of complaints from soldiers about their treatment by the new matron had to be answered by Vrooman in front of the board. He stated that Mary Ferguson treated the soldiers precisely the same as she treated the civilian patients. Dr. Procter, who recently had been appointed as a military medical officer, was asked to investigate. He reported that the matron's attitude to soldier-patients was "not satisfactory" and recommended some changes in her methods.

For their part, the soldier-patients continued to see themselves as distinct. The belief grew that they were different, not only from their fellow patients at the King Edward Sanatorium, but also from non-tubercular military patients at other hospitals. However, the disease from which they suffered accorded them no distinction. During the first nine months of 1917, 215 soldiers under the auspices of the Military Hospitals Commission died in Canadian hospitals; for 105 of them, the cause of death was tuberculosis.[9] In other words, the chief cause of death in the military population in Canada was the same as for the civilian population—tuberculosis.

The prolonged war strained hospital facilities and the military's administrative arrangements. In British Columbia, by the end of 1917, the thirty-two beds set aside for military patients at the King Edward Sanatorium were constantly in use, while the Balfour Sanatorium, intended for seventy patients, was accommodating 120. The Military Hospitals Commission made plans to construct a new facility for the treatment of tubercular military patients from British

Columbia, Alberta and Saskatchewan. Representatives of the MHC visited Kamloops in January 1918 to examine the Royal Inland Hospital and Tranquille as possible sites. At the same time, a reorganization saw the Military Hospitals Commission superseded by the Invalided Soldiers' Commission, which was placed under the Department of Soldiers' Civil Re-establishment (DSCR), a ministry of the federal government. The administrative changes did not alter the plans for a new facility and talks were held between the Invalided Soldiers' Commission and the British Columbia Anti-Tuberculosis Society.

The reaction of the Kamloops business community to the possibility of locating such an institution in the area contrasts sharply with its reaction of fifteen years earlier. Instead of reviving the Anti-Sanitarium (in Kamloops) League of 1904, the new Kamloops Chamber of Commerce, successor to the Inland Board of Trade, lobbied for the expansion. It announced in March that it planned to advertise "the health-giving qualities of Kamloops' climate from one end of the country to the other, and endeavour to make it a mecca for those seeking a mild and dry climate for many of the ills of humanity." In this, the Chamber of Commerce was supported by the recently amalgamated *Kamloops Standard-Sentinel* and the new *Kamloops Telegram*.[10] The fear of contagion and economic collapse of just a decade earlier found no public expression. Essentially, the community of Kamloops had returned to the boosterism of 1895, extolling the virtues of its location and climate, and welcoming to the area even those who suffered from the White Plague. When Dr. Irving opened his new Sunny View Sanatorium southwest of the city in 1915, the only newspaper comment was that a dozen such institutions would be of benefit to the community of Kamloops.[11]

The pro-Kamloops lobby would be needed. The Invalided Soldiers' Commission revised its plans and announced its intention to deal with treatment on a provincial basis. The British Columbia facility was to be constructed either at Tranquille or at the Experimental Farm near Penticton. The inevitable civic posturing took place, with advocates of the Penticton location particularly pointing out that the persistent dust storms at Tranquille inhibited the curative abilities of the institution. Boosters of the Tranquille site dismissed this criticism as exaggerated. Further discussions with the Anti-

Tuberculosis Society and Dr. Vrooman took place, and in May it was announced that Tranquille was to be the site of an extensive facility expected to cost $250,000. The provincial government would contribute $75,000 and the Department of Soldiers' Civil Re-establishment would cover all other construction costs. The facility was to become the property of the provincial government when it was no longer required for treatment of military patients. Tenders were called in August and, in late September, Charles Bentall's Dominion Construction Company of Vancouver began work on a three-storey infirmary and an adjacent service building.

Just as the tenders were called, Dr. Vrooman informed a surprised board of directors that he was resigning at the end of the year to take charge of the new Rotary Clinic in Vancouver. Vrooman would remain a director, but the disappointed board accepted his resignation with regret. During his eight years as superintendent, Vrooman had brought to the institution a sense of stability and continuity that managed to survive even the uncertain conditions brought about by the war in Europe. The last situation Dr. Vrooman had to face occurred with the influenza epidemic in the late autumn of 1918. He permitted no visitors and admitted no new patients from mid-October to mid-December, stating that the threat to the health of tubercular patients was too great. When he left to take up his responsibilities in Vancouver, not a single case of influenza had been reported at Tranquille.

Post-war Unrest

With the anticipated increase in military patients, it is not surprising that the search for Vrooman's replacement soon focussed on a man with experience in dealing with tubercular soldiers. Dr. Lester G. Houle, the medical superintendent of the Earl Grey Military Sanatorium in Regina, held the rank of captain in the Canadian army. Born at Charlottetown, Prince Edward Island, Houle had developed tuberculosis after graduating from McGill University. He was subsequently a patient and then an assistant for two years at Trudeau's sanatorium in Saranac, New York. He had been on the medical staff at Tranquille briefly in 1917 before taking charge of the Earl Grey Sanatorium. Mahon recommended his appointment, hoping in addition that the military would pay his salary, saving the board $3,600 annually. Those hopes were soon dissipated, but after a two-month trial as assistant superintendent, Houle was provisionally appointed to take charge of the institution in January 1919. The matron, recently married to patient Alexander Whitecross, hosted a social evening to welcome Dr. and Mrs. Houle and the new assistant superintendent, Dr. Busby—also a military man—to their new homes.

One of Houle's first recommendations to the board was that the institution should be renamed. The death of Edward VII, at a time of widespread hospital construction, and his support of medical causes generally and tuberculosis treatment in particular, had resulted in an abundance of institutions bearing his name throughout the British empire. This proliferation often caused confusion to doctors and the public, as well as to postal and shipping services. The board agreed with Houle's suggestion and, though there were criticisms that a name change would insult the memory of the late king, the institution reverted to its original name of Tranquille Sanatorium after March 1919. Officially, the Alexandra Ranch retained its name, but increasingly it was referred to as the Tranquille Ranch or Tranquille Farm.

At Tranquille, Houle did not inherit an easy situation. Inflation had become a serious problem during 1918, and the sanatorium returned to significant deficit situations in its operating accounts in 1918 and 1919. High wages elsewhere made it difficult to retain staff at a relatively isolated location like Tranquille and forced the society to raise the wages of its own staff in an attempt to do so. To assist with the management of the institution, Houle was given what Vrooman had so frequently requested when patient Alexander Whitecross became business manager in late 1919. Houle was thereby able to devote more time to medical matters. However, in relation to the soldiers, many matters were not purely medical. Most of the soldier patients were technically no longer soldiers due to new regulations of the DSCR, which henceforth would assume responsibility for invalid soldiers only after their discharge from the military. Nevertheless, the former soldiers continued to feel keenly the distinction between themselves and the other patients, despite the fact that they all now wore civilian clothes. Their difficulty in accepting the discipline required for treatment of their disease continued, and the stability required to enforce that discipline at

Tranquille was weakened when Mary Whitecross resigned in August 1919 to raise a family. She was replaced by assistant matron Jean White, who would also resign less than a year later in March 1920.

Houle, with his experience in the army and as superintendent of a military sanatorium, expected the obedience of those for whom he was responsible. He believed that it was best to treat soldiers as civilians, but at the Earl Grey institution in Regina, he was accustomed to a disciplinary system. He had there a disciplinary staff of a lieutenant and sergeant major and a guardroom that was used to sober up patients who had been on unauthorized binges. Even walks required supervision to keep patients away from the billiard halls and the other urban pleasures offered by downtown Regina. He anticipated at Tranquille to find less distraction by such temptations due to the isolation of the institution and therefore less discontent from patients at the restrictions on their activities.[12] At Tranquille, contrary to his expectations, he found considerable discontent, as soldier complaints about food and treatment were continuous.

At the same time, Houle was well aware that appropriate activities were essential for tubercular patients, and he welcomed all that the military had done to provide them. The Military Hospitals Commission loaned a moving picture projector and screen in January 1918, and movies were shown in the small auditorium of the Main Building for the benefit of all patients. Occupational therapy in carpentry and poultry raising was available after 1917, and a short five-hole golf course was laid out on the sand flats in front of the Main Building. The course was only usable in the late summer and fall when the water levels of the Thompson River were low, but it did provide a seasonal diversion for many. The patients' library, which had been growing slowly for many years, became a priority in anticipation of the one hundred additional patients expected in late 1919. Patient James Henderson, as unofficial librarian, took great care with the more than 1,300 volumes, and patient George Lothian printed postcards to raise funds for further purchases.

Expansion of the facility brought with it a number of concerns. The noise from the ongoing construction of the Infirmary and Service Building disrupted the peaceful atmosphere at Tranquille for many months. More troublesome to the board, however, were the anticipated long-term consequences of adding 102 patients to the existing population of the institution. Certainly, extra medical and non-medical staff would be required. The Infirmary was designed to accommodate the sanatorium's male support staff in the basement, but no new housing was available for the sixteen nurses the institution would soon require. Temporary plans were made to house all nurses on the third floor of the Infirmary, though this would reduce the number of beds available for patients. The board pressed the provincial government to match the offer of the DSCR to pay half the cost of a nurses' home and to loan the provincial government the other half.

Water supply and food supply also presented difficulties. The water supply was altered to provide a reservoir for fire protection and to eliminate the need for the water tower. The pumps now fed directly from the wells into the mains, but the water supply was generally felt to be inadequate and excessively alkaline. The food requirements of the expanded institution could not be met by the Alexandra Ranch. The society's hope that it could acquire the Cooney Ranch was frustrated by the fact that it was still not for sale, even after the death of Charles Cooney in 1917. There was no money to make the purchase anyway. A proposal from the Kamloops House Committee in August 1919 that the society acquire the Austin Farm, eight miles north of Kamloops on the North Thompson River, was also rejected by the board. Quite clearly, the society simply lacked the financial ability to make the purchase. The board knew that the additional money for wages, supplies, building and alterations could come only from the provincial government, especially when the number of military patients began to decline in a few years time. Both levels of government were presented with financial requests. The DSCR was asked to increase its payments for soldier patients from $1.50 per day to $2 per day; the provincial government was asked again to take over responsibility for Tranquille.[13]

Though the new buildings would not be ready for occupation until December, they were officially opened on the afternoon of 6 October 1919. In the excitement of the occasion, there came together at Tranquille many of the figures who had played prominent roles in the institution. Major Dr. Arthur Procter, who as the medical officer

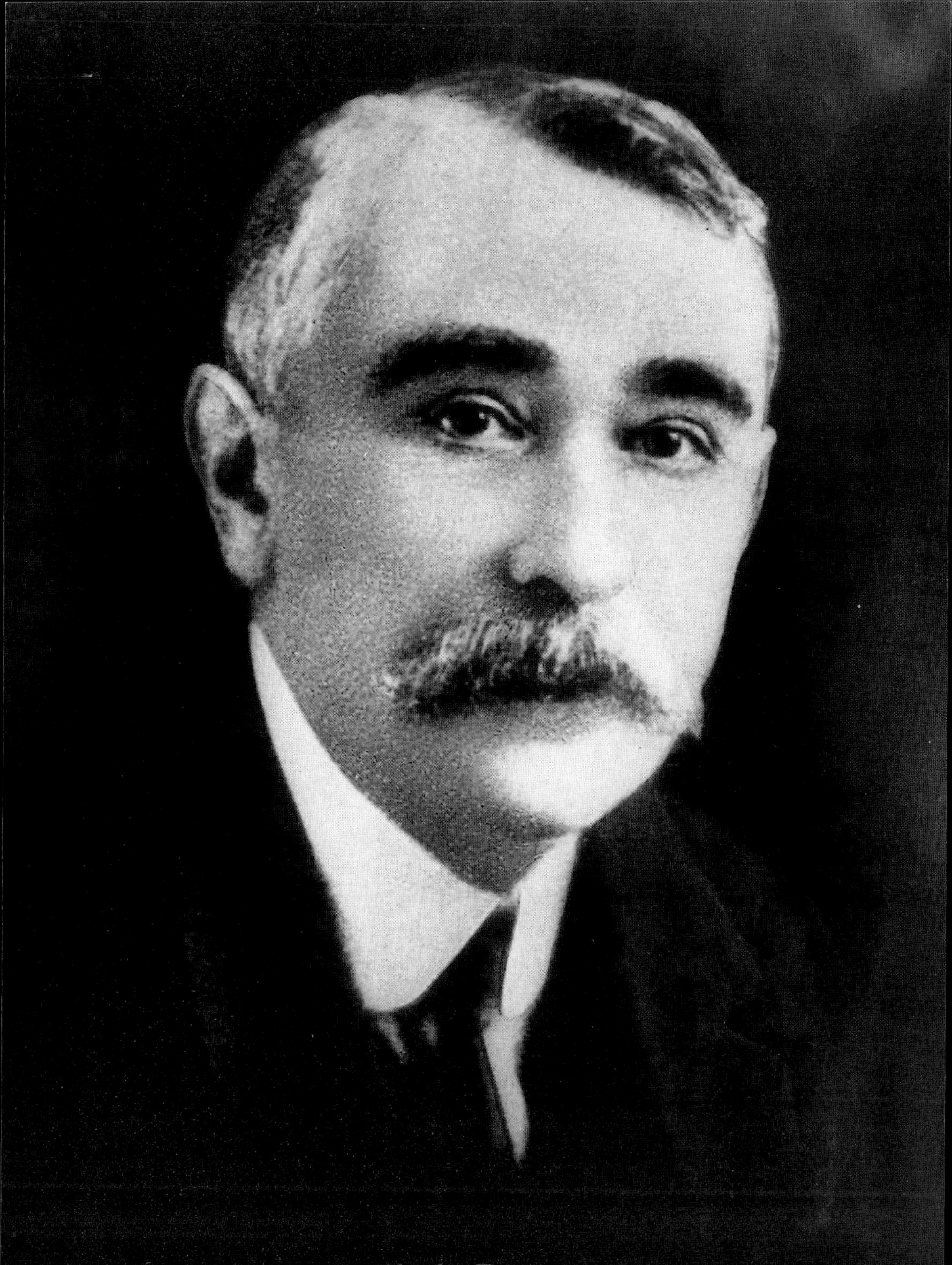

Dr. Charles Fagan
(Courtesy BCARS A - 02133)

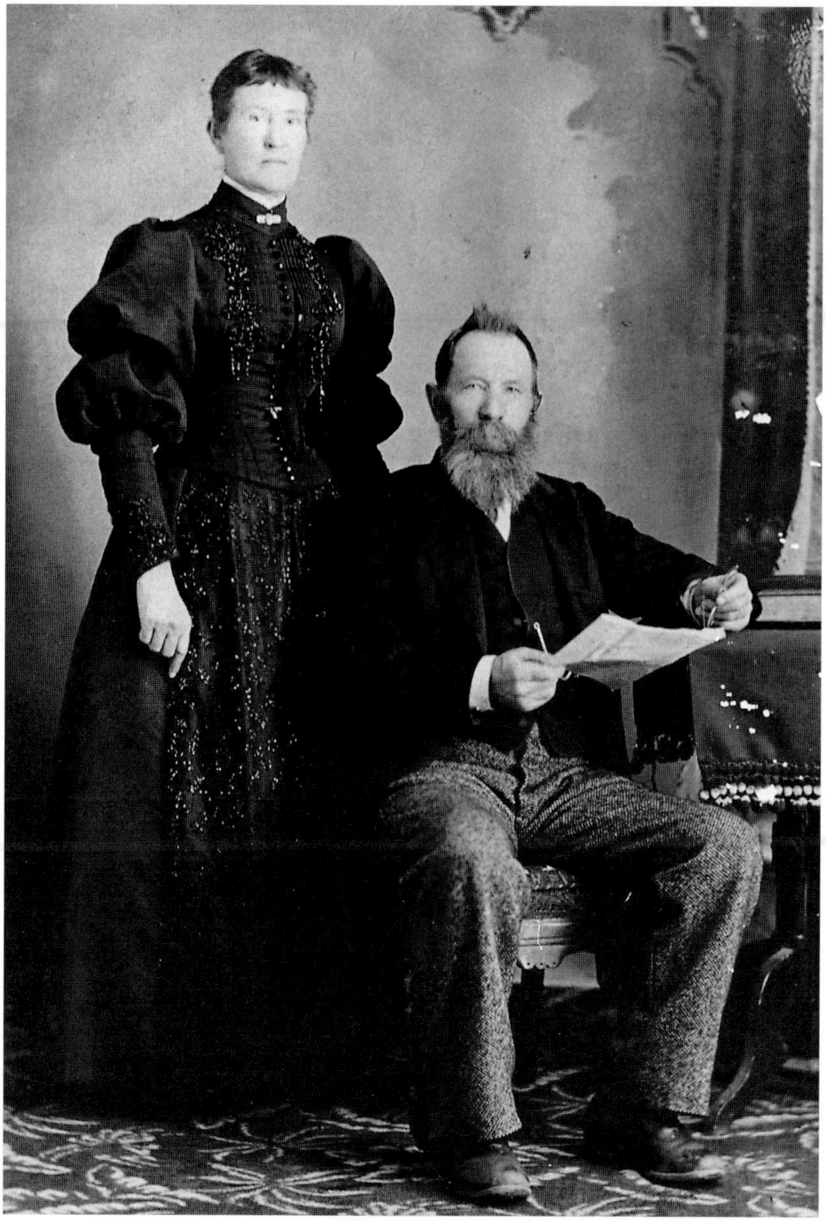

Jane and William Fortune
(Courtesy KMA 284)

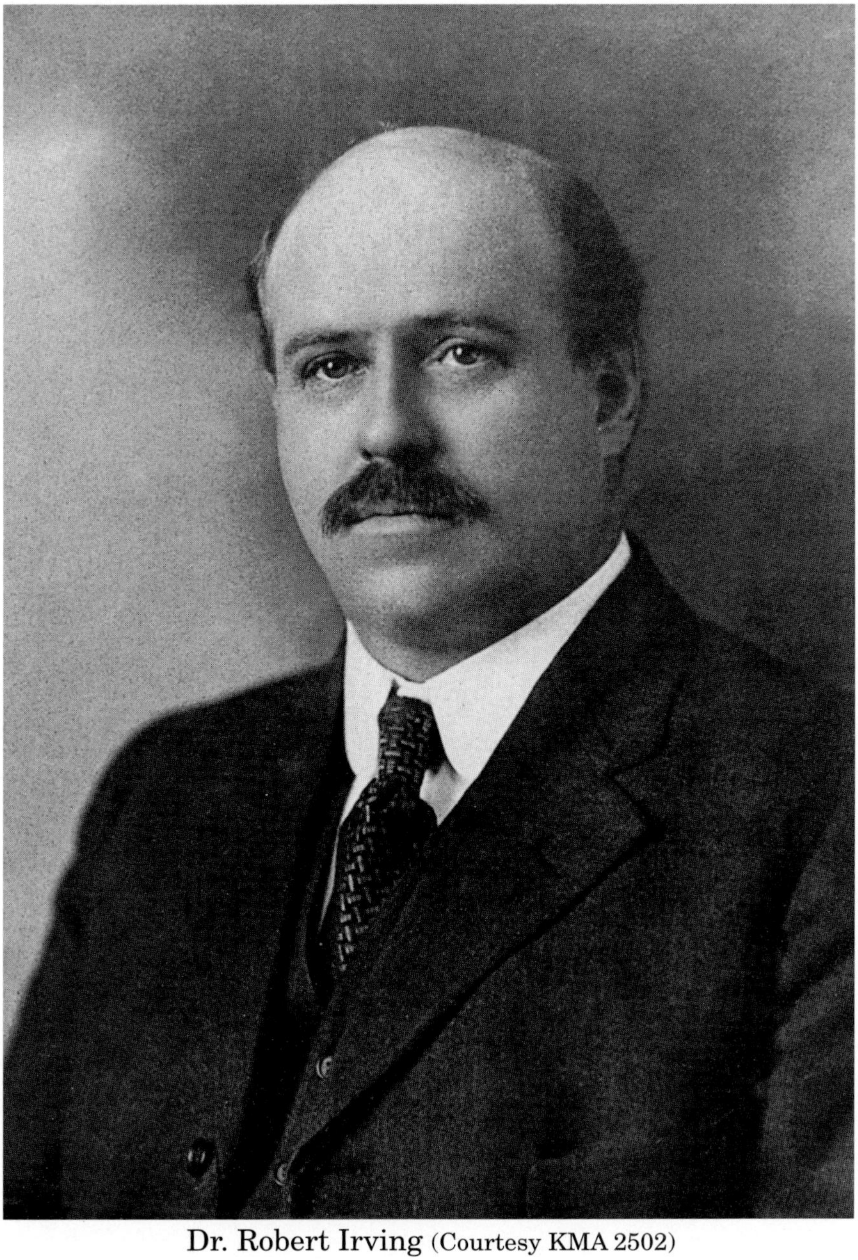

Dr. Robert Irving (Courtesy KMA 2502)

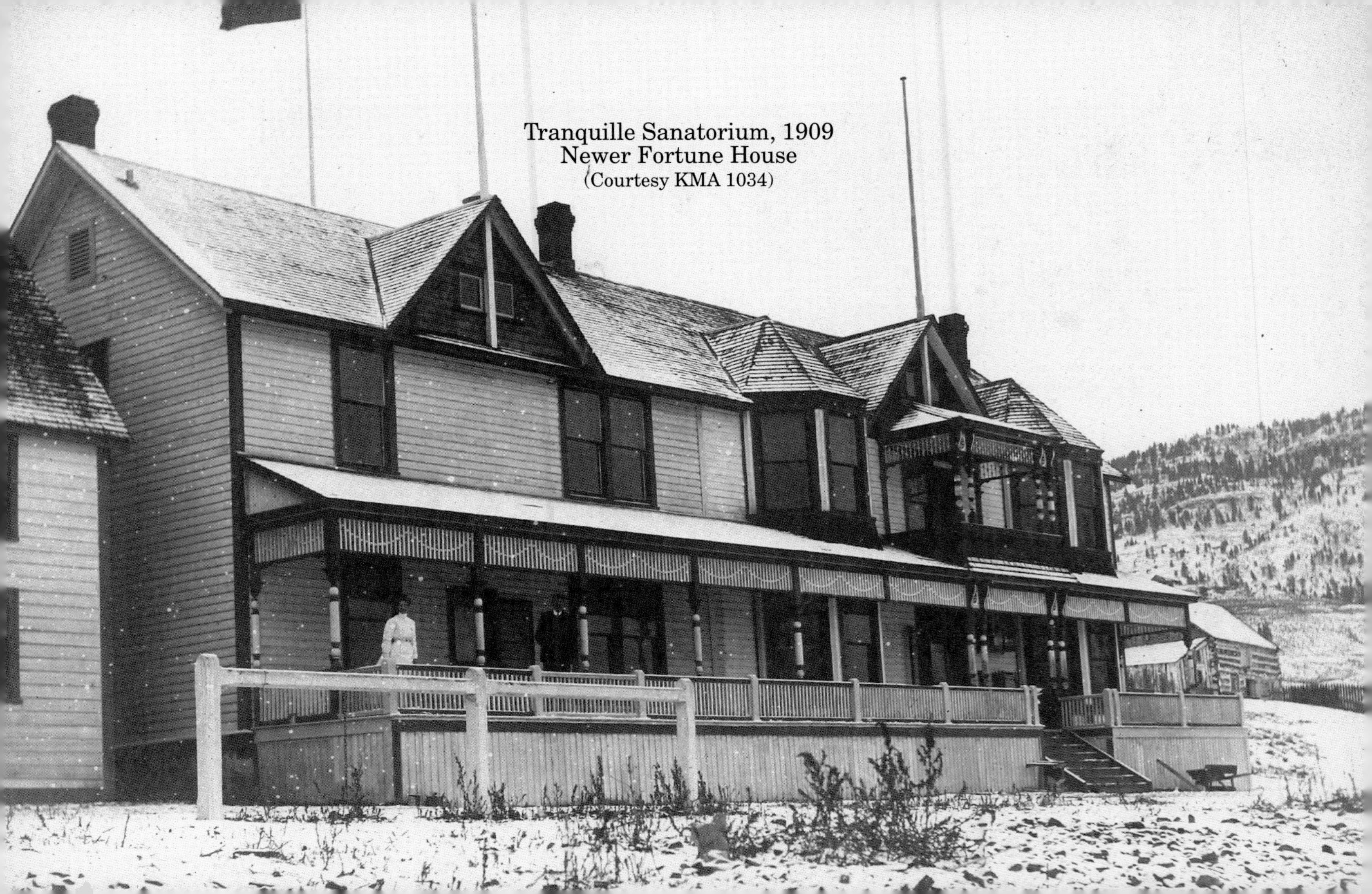

Tranquille Sanatorium, 1909
Newer Fortune House
(Courtesy KMA 1034)

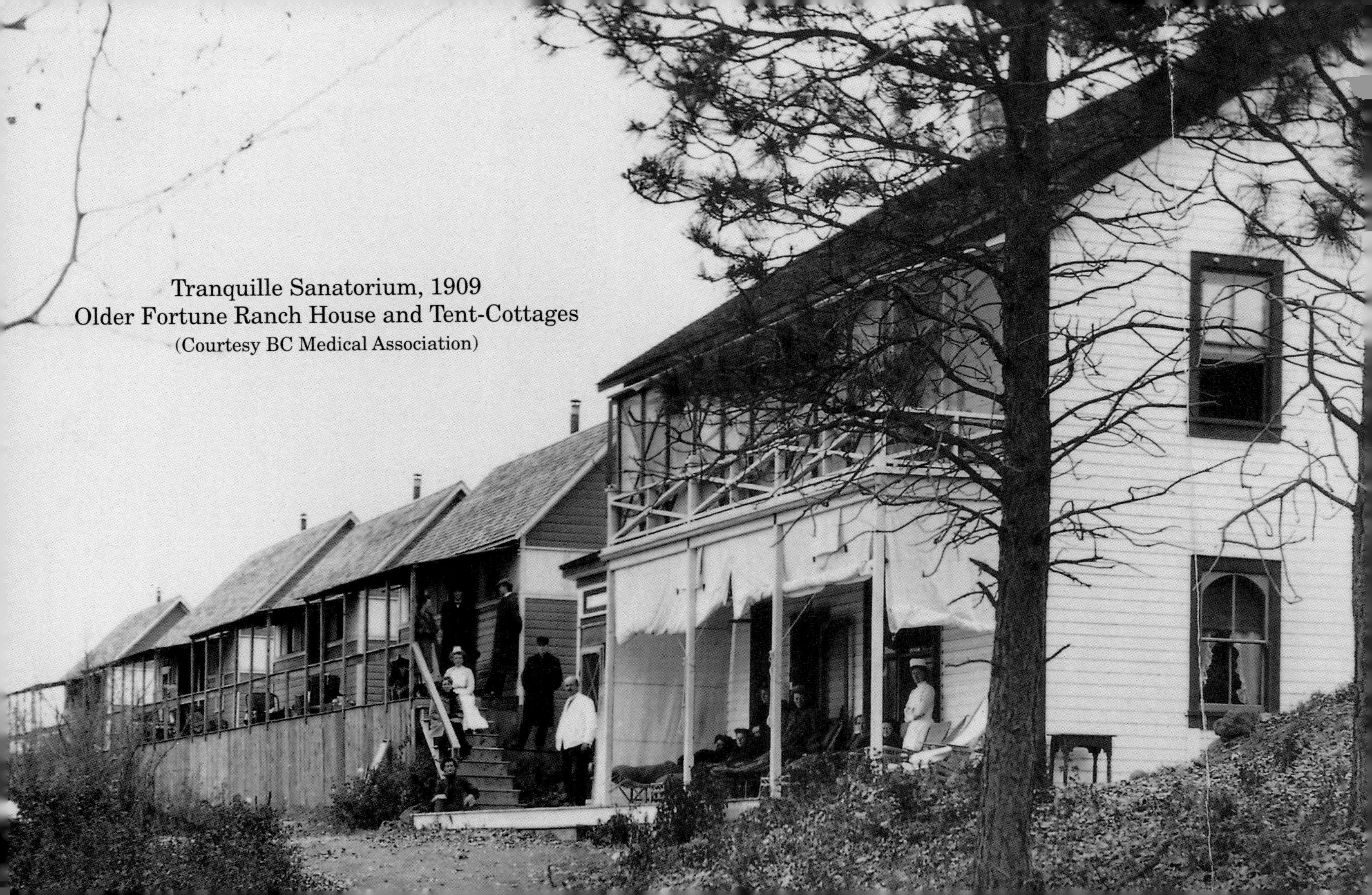

Tranquille Sanatorium, 1909
Older Fortune Ranch House and Tent-Cottages
(Courtesy BC Medical Association)

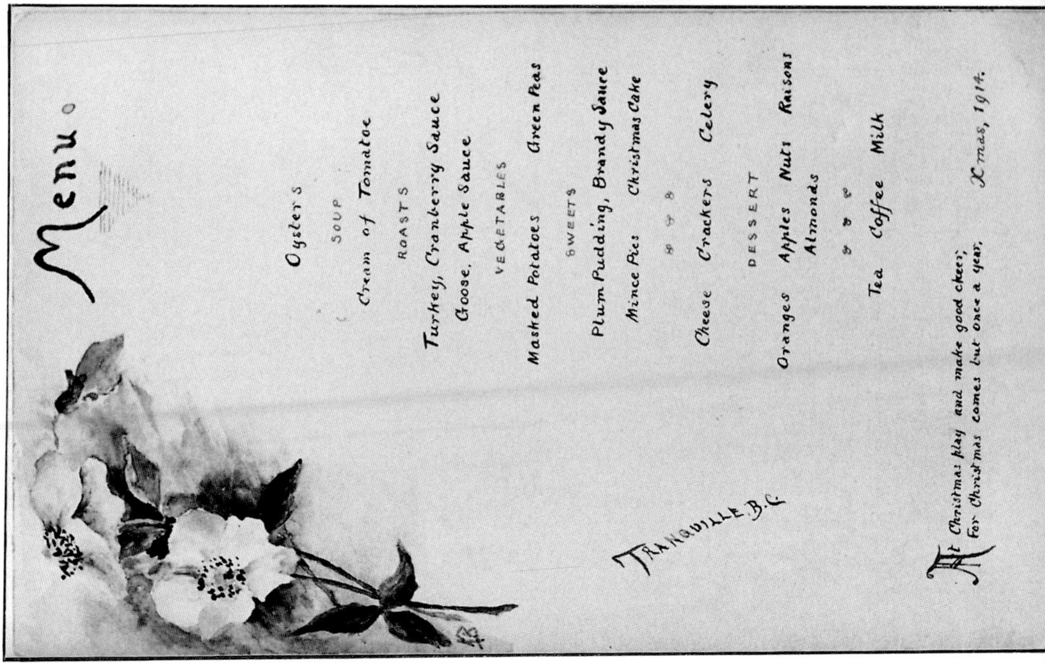

Menu

Oysters

SOUP

Cream of Tomatoe

ROASTS

Turkey, Cranberry Sauce

Goose, Apple Sauce

VEGETABLES

Mashed Potatoes   Green Peas

SWEETS

Plum Pudding, Brandy Sauce

Mince Pies   Christmas Cake

Cheese   Crackers   Celery

DESSERT

Oranges   Apples   Nuts   Raisons

Almonds

Tea   Coffee   Milk

At Christmas play and make good cheer;
For Christmas comes but once a year.

Xmas, 1914.

Tranquille B.C.

Christmas Dinner Menu, 1914
(Courtesy BC Lung Association)

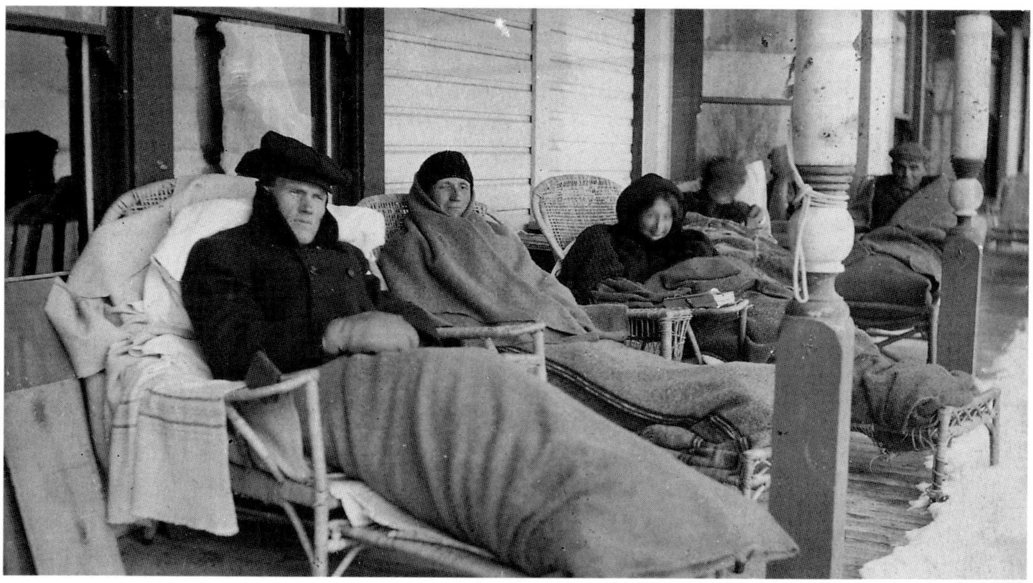

The Fresh Air Cure at -34° F
(Courtesy KMA 4341)

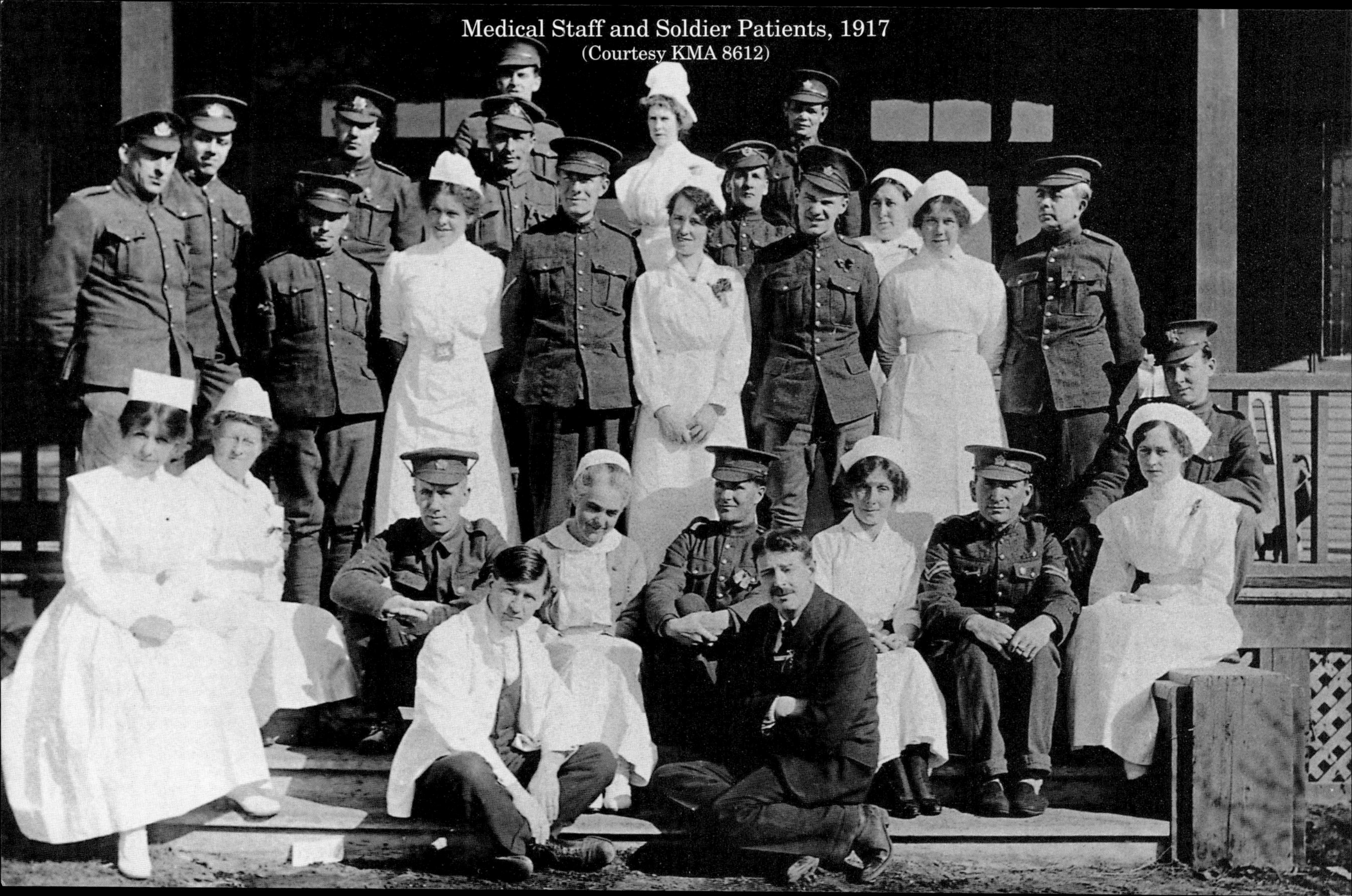

Medical Staff and Soldier Patients, 1917
(Courtesy KMA 8612)

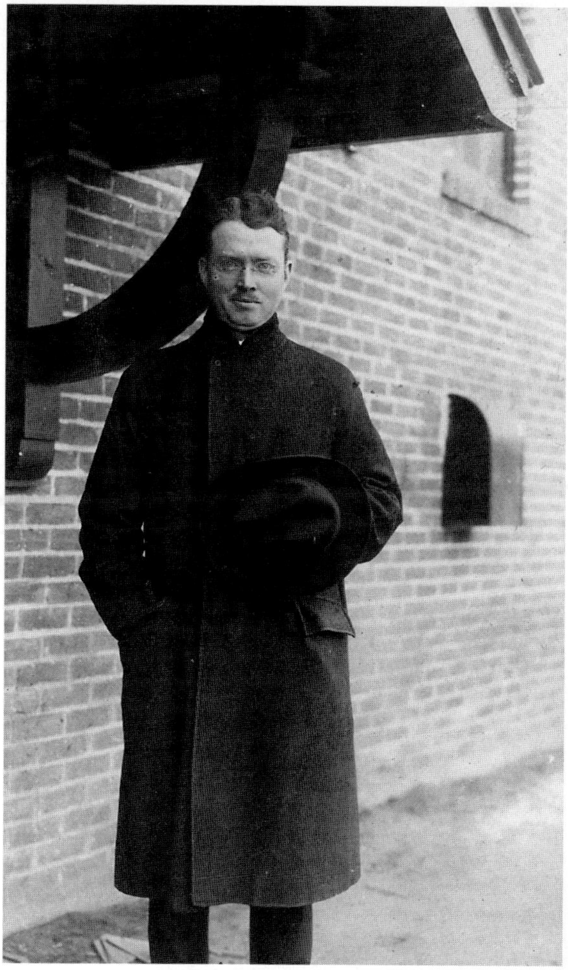

Dr. Lester Houle
(Courtesy KMA 8688)

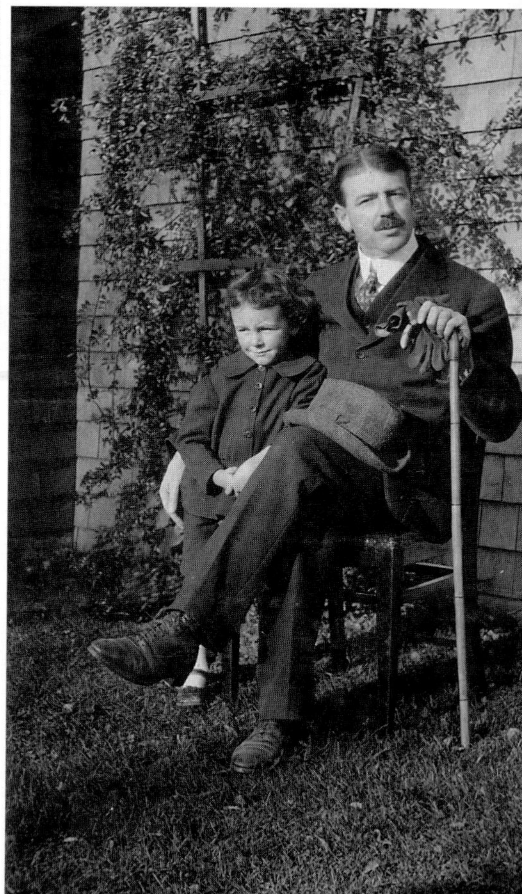

Dr. Charles Vrooman
(Courtesy KMA 8686)

of Royal Inland Hospital in 1901 had so strongly favoured the establishment of a sanatorium locally, represented the DSCR. Dr. Vrooman arrived with nearly four dozen members of the Vancouver Board of Trade. Dr. Houle proudly conducted tours of the new buildings, while Strachan just as proudly showed people around the ranch. Chairman of the board of directors Edward Mahon, society president C.H. Gatewood and other members of the society were present, but the honour of officially opening the facility went to Susan Wood, longtime president of the very active Kamloops branch society. One newspaper reporter noted that, with the addition of the new structures, Tranquille had become “a fine pile o’ buildings.”

The Invalided Soldiers’ Commission had paid for the Infirmary, the Service Building, electrical and plumbing requirements, alterations to the powerhouse, and an underground tunnel connecting the Service Building to the powerhouse. A garage, x-ray equipment, and operating rooms were also added. Only the proposed nurses’ home had been cut from the original construction plans. Changes in the racial composition of the labour force also occurred. A new steam laundry replaced the Chinese hand laundry, while Chinese workers were also eliminated from the kitchen. More than ten years after it had first been enunciated, Irving’s desire for an all-white labour force had been achieved. Apart from a few Native ranch hands and a few soldier-patients, Tranquille after 1919 reflected the prevailing racial attitudes of the province, with an effective colour bar in effect for both patients and staff.

Federal expenditure on the project amounted to over $300,000, while the province provided $75,000 as promised. Assistant Superintendent Busby entertained and instructed guests by stepping in front of the x-ray machine to “present an interior view of himself.” In his formal speech, Mahon stated that daily milk requirements would rise from sixty gallons to 100, and that a nurses’ home was desperately needed. He remarked upon the “liberality of the Dominion authorities” and took the opportunity to renew the call for a provincial takeover of the institution.[14]

That call soon received much support when it was realized that the society’s obligation was to provide acute care to 102 military patients in the new building and to as many as sixty military patients suffering an incipient form of the disease in the two pavilions. In other words, though the capacity of the institution had increased to 230 patients, the beds available to civilian patients could be reduced to only seventy. In a province where rates of tuberculosis infection were still rising, this caused an outcry that was muted only by the prevailing attitude that soldiers deserved the consideration of a grateful nation. The *Victoria Times* responded to the society's announcement that Tranquille could accept no more civilian patients by saying that "without the help of the state," few in British Columbia could take advantage of the great promise of the cure offered by the dry belt and Tranquille.[15]

The Tranquillian

Just six months after his appointment, Dr. Houle helped to establish what would prove to be the institution's most enduring and most successful vehicle for public education and fundraising. H.R. Farmer, formerly an employee of the *Vancouver Province*, suggested to Houle that a monthly publication for sanatorium residents could combine news of interest to residents with educational articles about the nature of tuberculosis care. Houle lent the project his full support. Farmer recruited a small team of interested patients, while Houle contacted prospective contributors on medical topics. After printing arrangements were made with the *Kamloops Telegram*, the first four-page issue of *The Tranquillian* appeared on 1 August 1919. The first issue featured an appreciation by Dr. Procter of the work of Dr. Fagan, and an article by Houle on the history and treatment of tuberculosis. Subsequent issues would all include comparable didactic material, and the publication would soon proclaim in the masthead of each issue that it was "Published for the Education of the Well and in the Interests of the Sick." However, the attraction for sanatorium residents was the increasing amount of news of patients, former patients, activities upcoming, and activities past.

Photographs of picnic groups and of the boats at the sanatorium dock are interspersed with reports of fishing expeditions to Trout Lake and corn roasts on the beach of Kamloops Lake enjoyed by both staff and ambulant patients. When Walter Hillam, another patient with newspaper experience, took over editorial responsibilities in June 1920, he appealed to residents for articles and short stories. Many of the submissions he received had a distinct political tone, especially those from the soldier population. The periodical was adopted by the fledgling Invalided Tubercular Soldiers Welfare League as its official organ, and the affairs of veterans and a proposed tuberculosis colony on the Kamloops Indian Reserve received much attention. Politics was not confined to veterans' issues: the entire text of an open letter to provincial politicians concerning tuberculosis treatment was printed in December 1920. Many contributors chose pseudonyms indicating their status as patients. Articles appeared by A. Lunger and regular contributor Ah Bum Lung.

Other submissions, such as this parody of Hamlet's famous soliloquy, made light of the medical condition that had brought them all—civilians, soldiers, medical staff, and non-medical staff—to Tranquille:

> T. B. or not T. B.—that is the question:
> Whether 'tis nobler, in the mind to suffer
> The pains and trials of tuberculosis,
> Or to take shelter in a T.B. San.,
> And by much "chasing" end them?
> To chase—to rest—to sleep—
> To eat; and thus to try to end
> The heartaches and the thousand shocks
> That T. B.'s flesh is heir to—'tis a consummation
> Devoutly to be reached. To rest—to sleep—to eat
> To sleep! Perchance to snore! Ay, there's the rub;
> For in this life of ours, alas!—what noises come
> When we, imprisoned in our narrow cells,
> Must live and listen all the long, long hours:
> 'Tis this and more that makes
> Calamity of life at Tranquille.
> For who would bear the sighs, and snores, and coughs,
> The nurse's wrath, the doctor's contumely,
> The pangs of idleness, the long delay,
> The official "tyranny," the penalties imposed,
> The cold roast beef, the solitary walks...[16]

Poetry quickly became one of the most popular features of the publication.

Because so little has survived elsewhere concerning the day to day life of Tranquille residents, even the newspaper's brief mention of individual patients and staff, of picnics and performances are of considerable interest. For example, an election of sorts is recorded for the first time in January 1920. Perhaps a soldier-patient innovation, the comic election became an annual event, with an unofficial mayor decided by patient voting. Reports on the year-end concerts by the students of Tranquille School identify several Cooney and Strachan children as students. A Civilian Comforts Committee was established by patients, perhaps to ensure that veteran patients did not receive all the attention of the philanthropic community. With the financial success of *The Tranquillian* and with donations from the branch societies so sharply curtailed, profits from the sale of the newspaper were soon earmarked to provide necessities for poorer patients. Under the direction of the medical superintendent and the matron, the Civilian Comforts Committee quickly became the body through which clothing and other necessities were supplied to indigent patients.

A Society Nearing Exhaustion

Acknowledging more overtly that it was overwhelmed by its responsibilities, the board in January 1920 decided to seek a takeover by petitioning the provincial government. The election that was called at this time provided an opportunity to lay the question before the voters and the political parties. In an open letter to Premier John Oliver and Opposition Leader W.J. Bowser, Mahon pointed out the current problems of civilian waiting lists, lack of accommodation (especially for nurses), and the need for more money for building and operation. He stated bluntly that it was impossible for the society to continue under current financial arrangements and asked each leader to state party policy on the question of tuberculosis treatment. He received only the customary general statements of support for the society's work, and was disappointed that the issue did not become a factor in the election campaign.

Nevertheless, it was soon after the Liberals' re-election that reports began to appear suggesting that the government was about to assume responsibility for the Tranquille Sanatorium. Though still apparently somewhat reluctant, the provincial government nevertheless was finally involved in serious discussions with the society about a takeover. The negotiations were not easy. In July, a dispirited board learned the government wanted the inclusion of the Greaves legacy as a condition of the takeover. The society had intended to continue its work using the Greaves bequest, but over the objections of Dr. Vrooman, agreed to the stipulation. The September 1920 issue of *The Tranquillian* reported that a takeover was imminent and approved of the development editorially. Frustrated at how long the process was taking, the society nevertheless prepared to wind up its affairs.

As they did so, they were forced to deal with rapidly deteriorating conditions at Tranquille. The mortgage still due on the Fortune ranch came up for renewal and no bank would take it. Finally, at eight percent interest, the mortgage was accepted privately by North Kamloops resident Francis Morant. Significant salary increases were granted to most staff during 1918-20, largely to ensure that sufficient personnel were retained to operate the institution. By the end of 1920, nurses' wages, for example, were double what they had been in 1914. Though the salaries of the new senior medical staff remained stable, ranch manager Strachan and business manager Whitecross received significant increases. Accommodation difficulties multiplied. The basement of the new Infirmary proved to be insufferably hot. Consequently, to house temporarily the male employees of the sanatorium, the bunk houses put up by Dominion Construction for the use of its workers were purchased at a cost of $1,000. No money was available for a nurses' home or any other building as the provincial government contemplated its takeover, so nurses continued to occupy the third floor of the Infirmary. Edward Mahon, after a visit to Tranquille in May 1920, informed the board:

> There is a constant flow up and down the C.N.R. of Nurses, Chefs, Cooks, Orderleys [sic], etc. With the salaries obtainable elsewhere and the uncomfortable conditions at Tranquille, it makes the management at the Institution almost impossible.[17]

Significant as these problems were, they were not the main reason for Mahon's investigative visit. Many new complaints had been received from soldier-patients about a variety of issues, and a widespread revolt against the authority of the superintendent was taking place. The complaints focussed on the familiar issues of quality of food and the expectation that able patients should make their beds and keep their rooms clean. The rebels threatened that if a single soldier-patient were expelled for non-cooperation in these matters, all would leave the institution immediately. Though the revolt was essentially over by mid-June, Houle acknowledged that five were "still on strike." Complaining that his authority was undermined by the DSCR's inability to force those under its auspices to follow institutional discipline, Houle tendered his resignation. Whether the resignation was sought by the board or whether it was unanticipated is unclear. Perhaps Houle simply wanted the board's endorsement of his actions in his disputes with soldier-patients. If so, he must have been surprised when the board accepted the resignation, stating that a change of management would "be to the benefit of all concerned." Houle departed towards the end of August to enter private practice in Kamloops with Dr. Burris.[18]

The society's financial concerns were eased somewhat as the DSCR agreed to pay half the salary of the new superintendent, but the search for a suitable choice ran into trouble immediately. The board's preferred candidate, Dr. R.J. Collins, had been a patient at Balfour before he joined the medical staff there. Ironically, the Balfour Sanatorium had just experienced a serious soldier-patient strike over their opposition to the DSCR's decision to close the institution and move remaining patients to Tranquille. However, Collins declined the position at the last moment due to renewed concern about his health, and Dr. Vrooman spent the last week of August at Tranquille as acting superintendent. James Kearney of the Tranquille medical staff and, briefly, Kamloops doctor A.E.H. Bennett alternated as acting superintendents while the search was conducted. Dr. Collins then re-accepted the position, but his appointment was not confirmed as negotiations with the provincial government continued. The government wanted to make its own selection of the man to run the institution it was about to acquire. Dr. Kearney, therefore, was offered in November a three-month appointment, which was later extended. The last disgruntled patients from Balfour arrived in December, bringing to thirty the number transferred from the Kootenay institution. Kearney was relieved to report that no further discipline problems were occurring.

Finally, in February 1921, with little discernible enthusiasm on either side, the provincial government and the British Columbia Anti-Tuberculosis Society signed their agreement. On 17 March, Provincial Secretary John McLean rose in the legislature to introduce the bill to enable the provincial government to take over Tranquille. His speech included statistics revealing much about the government support of the institution over the years. Whereas the Conservative administration from 1907 to 1917 had expended an average of $28,000 annually at Tranquille, the average annual expenditure during the four years of Liberal rule had risen to more than $70,000. The assets of the society, comprising essentially the land and buildings at Tranquille in addition to the Greaves legacy, amounted to $785,935. Liabilities totalled $53,000, with $20,000 still owed on the mortgage and the remainder due to a variety of creditors. The 119 soldier patients at Tranquille continued to be maintained by the DSCR, but the monthly deficit in the operating account nevertheless stood at about $1,500 at the time of the takeover. In explaining the reasons for the government decision, McLean confirmed what some members of the Anti-Tuberculosis Society had maintained since 1904. He said the takeover was necessary because it had become "too large and important an undertaking to be managed and supported by voluntary effort, and, secondly because the care of contagious disease of this nature should be the duty of the province."[19] The *Tranquille Sanatorium Agreement Ratification Act* received a quick passage. The government was to take over the operation at Tranquille, assuming all board assets and liabilities, on 1 April 1921.

A relieved board met for the last time on 31 March. Letters of thanks were prepared for the society's secretary, the House Committee in Kamloops, and the surviving women's auxiliaries. Only the New Westminster branch and the nominally active Vancouver branch actually remained to be advised officially that their services would be required no longer. The Kamloops branch in December 1920 had dissolved to merge with the local Red Cross organization, intending to carry on its work at Tranquille under the Red Cross umbrella. The board's fourteenth and final report for the year 1920 was not completed. It would have revealed many difficulties, many unhappy creditors, and an operating deficit of nearly $20,000.

With the government takeover of Tranquille, the British Columbia Anti-Tuberculosis Society finally got what it had been asking for. In that there was some consolation. However, the conclusion of the affairs of the society can have brought little joy to its members. As an exercise in private philanthropy, the organization had overcome many obstacles (including its own excessive optimism) and had persevered long enough to show a reluctant provincial government where its duty properly lay. However, the society had been unable to operate the institution it founded in the manner it had intended—as a sanatorium for incipient cases of tuberculosis. During the nearly fourteen years of the society's operation of the sanatorium, more than 1,700 victims of tuberculosis—the majority in advanced stages of the disease—were cared for at Tranquille. Even so, the organization received only token acknowledgements of its achievement from the government and newspapers as its responsibilities concluded.

Chapter Notes

1 British Columbia Lung Association Archives, box 1, W.H. Hatfield, "A History of Tuberculosis in British Columbia, Part I."
2 National Archives of Canada (NAC), RG 38, volume 287, Military Hospitals Commission, Report by E.H. Scammell, 15 December 1916.
3 NAC, RG 38, volume 287 Military Hospitals Commission, Minutes, 15 December 1915.
4 University of British Columbia (UBC), Records of the British Columbia Anti-Tuberculosis Society, Minute Book, 12 September 1916.
5 NAC RG 38, volume 287, Military Hospitals Commission, Minutes 8 September 1916; Report by E.H. Scammell 15 December 1916; Desmond Morton and Glenn Wright, *Winning the Second Battle: Canadian Veterans and the Return to Civilian Life, 1915-1930* (Toronto, 1987) p. 35.
6 UBC, Records of the British Columbia Anti-Tuberculosis Society, Minute Book, 23 August 1916.
7 Tenth Report of the British Columbia Anti-Tuberculosis Society, pp. 8-11.
8 *Vancouver Province*, 6 December 1917.
9 NAC, RG 38, volume 287, Military Hospitals Commission, Memoranda and Reports, 1916-1920, 7 November 1917.
10 *Kamloops Standard-Sentinel*, 25 January 1918, 8 March 1918; Telegram, 7 March 1918, p. 2.
11 *Inland Sentinel*, 1 November 1915, p. 3.
12 NAC RG 38, volume 371, Military Hospitals Commission, Captain L.G. Houle, "The Problem of the Tuberculous Soldier in Saskatchewan," Care of Tuberculous Soldiers Bulletin No. 8 (28 February 1918).
13 UBC, Records of the British Columbia Anti-Tuberculosis Society, Minutes, 31 July 1919 and 28 August 1919.
14 *Kamloops Standard-Sentinel*, 7 October 1919; *Vancouver World*, 8 October 1919; *Vancouver Province*, 8 October 1919.
15 *Victoria Times*, reprinted in *Kamloops Standard-Sentinel*, 7 November 1919, p. 7.
16 This and the rest of former patient V.A.L.'s tribute to Shakespeare and tuberculosis can be found in *The Tranquillian*, October 1920, p. 1.
17 UBC, Records of the British Columbia Anti-Tuberculosis Society, Minute Book, Report to Board of Directors by Edward Mahon, n.d.
18 UBC, Records of the British Columbia Anti-Tuberculosis Society Minute book, 24 June 1920. Dr. Houle worked in Kamloops until 1923 when his own tuberculosis returned. He entered the Manitoba Sanatorium in Ninette where he died in 1925.
19 *Vancouver Province*, 17 March 1921.

A Separate World: 1921-1937

The transition from private to public ownership went smoothly, at least partly because all senior staff employed by the British Columbia Anti-Tuberculosis Society remained in their positions. Acting medical superintendent James Kearney, Matron J.A. Morrice, and ranch superintendent David Strachan became employees of the provincial government on 1 April 1921. Approximately one hundred employees, in addition to senior medical staff and the ranch manager, found themselves on the provincial payroll. Though the employment crisis did not end, it had eased considerably by the time of the takeover, as inflationary pressures were diminishing sharply. When, after considerable deliberation, the government announced the selection of its first medical superintendent in early November, Dr. Kearney left Tranquille to pursue graduate studies in chest diseases, while both Morrice and Strachan continued in their positions. As the institution prepared to welcome the new superintendent, the uncertainties associated with the private institution were forgotten. Quite abruptly, stability seemed to replace instability.

Alexander Lapp graduated from Toronto Medical School in 1916 before seeing military service. He had experience at the Muskoka Sanitarium and, for the previous three years, had been assistant superintendent at the Sainte Agathe des Monts Sanatorium near Montreal. On 9 November 1921, he began what would prove to be a long association with the Tranquille Sanatorium. Though not quite thirty years of age at the time of his appointment, Lapp soon demonstrated that he would be able to provide additional stability to the institution as a capable administrator.

Considering the potential for further soldier unrest, the provincial authorities undoubtedly expected that the new superintendent would be able to maintain order. Dr. Lapp did not disappoint them. He made it understood that the rules and regulations of the institution were not open for discussion and negotiation. He took steps to discourage social contact between patients and employees, as well as contact between medical and non-medical staff. Essentially, he sought to establish not just order, but a pre-war order where social distinctions were clear and unchallenged by the forces of change that the Great War had unleashed. Though he did not achieve these objectives quickly or without resultant difficulties, they were all accomplished over time.

More Soldiers, More Politics

By the time of Dr. Lapp's appointment, the soldier population had already begun to decline. Just six months earlier, at the time of the takeover by the provincial government, the soldiers at the institution were sufficiently numerous that the Tranquille Sanatorium could have been legitimately regarded as a military hospital. Of the 210 patients under treatment on 1 April 1921, 119 were being maintained by the Department of Soldiers' Civil Re-establishment (DSCR). In other words, the civilian patient population in 1921 was no greater than it had been after the opening of the Main Building in 1909. The military presence also dramatically affected the ratio of males to females. Of 179 patients admitted during the course of the first year of government operation, only nineteen were female. What was not affected was the average age and medical condition of the patients: most were between the ages of sixteen and forty-five, and most were in advanced stages of the disease.[1] Though the numbers of soldiers would decline slowly over the years and though the number of women patients would gradually rise, the tone of the institution—male and military—would long be retained. By 1922, however, there were sufficient women patients to require a separate building to accommodate them. The Main Building was designated for their use, leaving the Infirmary, the two pavilions and the shacks for male occupation. From this time forward, a stricter segregation of the sexes was maintained.

The soldier-patients continued to be strong advocates for their own welfare. As early as 1918, branches of the Invalided Tubercular Soldiers Welfare League (ITSWL) were established at almost all sanatoria in Canada. According to some reports, the league originated at Tranquille. The purpose of the ITSWL was made clear by its name, and the publication of *The Tranquillian* in August 1919 provided an opportunity to publicize the league's goals and activities. *The Tranquillian* was adopted as the official organ of the league in

February 1920. In response to ITSWL pressure, the federal government appointed the Board of Tuberculosis Consultants to report on the care and rehabilitation of tubercular soldiers. League members at Tranquille made presentations to members of the task force when a delegation visited the sanatorium in early July 1920 and to Prime Minister Arthur Meighen when he visited in October.

Part of the presentations to both the Board of Tuberculosis Consultants and to Prime Minister Meighen was a proposal that would generate controversy for years to come. Kamloops resident and Chamber of Commerce employee Henry Denison had proposed as early as 1916 that the Kamloops Indian Band be relocated at the Harper Ranch north of Mount Paul. This would allow the five thousand acres directly opposite Kamloops to be made available to develop a model community for disabled veterans. The scheme echoed a popular perception in Kamloops that a greater distance between the settler community and the Native population would not only enhance the business prospects of the city, but also somehow benefit the Indian Band as well. Supporters of the proposal to move the reserve could now add patriotism to their arguments. By the end of the war, Denison was more specifically proposing that the model village should be for tubercular veterans. In June 1920, three members of the ITSWL visited Denison in Kamloops to discuss the scheme. In July, the Kamloops branch of the Great War Veterans' Association adopted a resolution calling on the federal government to appropriate the Kamloops Indian Reserve to establish a model village for tubercular veterans. Denison then published a pamphlet on the subject, claiming the scheme had the support of many organizations, the provincial government, and the prime minister. The pamphlet summarized the scheme:

> Briefly, the plan as presented to the federal government calls for a city specially designed for the cure of tuberculosis, where our afflicted men—single or with families—could reside under the most healthful and happy surroundings, in homes with small plots of various sizes, thus securing the benefits of the country with the comforts of city life. The plan also calls for an industrial site; business and residential sections; parks;

> in fact a combination of most modern plans for a GARDEN CITY.

He defended the plan against the charge of extravagance by arguing that the "best is none too good for those who have suffered for the Empire's sake."[2]

The ITSWL expanded on the proposal in its presentations to the prime minister and the Board of Tuberculosis Consultants. A village containing light manufacturing shops in airy structures was to be established for a workforce of veterans capable of working reduced shifts of two to six hours in pottery, boot-making and furniture construction. Agricultural holdings would surround the village. *The Tranquillian*, under the editorship of ITSWL member Walter Hillam at the time, editorially supported the proposal, as did the *Vancouver World*. No mention was made in either the presentations or the editorials of what the attitude of the Kamloops Indian Band might be to the proposal.[3]

The scheme was receiving local attention when the Tranquille Sanatorium was taken over by the provincial government in April 1921. The federal election at the end of the year gave it further exposure, as local Conservatives Henry Denison, Robert Irving and lawyer Frederick Fulton saw an opportunity to gain local support for their party. Irving gave the scheme his unqualified endorsement and advised the minister of the interior, R.J. Manion, in September that the proposal had "almost universal support" in the Kamloops area. He noted that "cured" patients from the sanatorium, upon release, usually suffered a recurrence of the disease when they returned to employment. He advised Manion that Denison's scheme offered a "wonderful opportunity" to avoid these breakdowns. Fulton also contacted Manion in support of the proposal.[4]

A serious discussion of the proposal occurred at a meeting of the DSCR in Ottawa in 1921. The meeting heard the opinion of one participant that agricultural produce from a tuberculosis colony was not likely to sell well. Another made the remark that "practically everyone around Kamloops is tuberculous anyway." A third noted that the Department of Indian Affairs had "absolutely discouraged" any further consideration of the proposal to move the Indian population.[5]

However, the proponents of the scheme in Kamloops were not discouraged and pressed the new federal Liberal administration for action on the matter. When the deputy minister of Indian Affairs declared that local opposition to the scheme was widespread, Kamloops city manager A.S. Fraser replied that when he investigated the claim, he found few opposed. Ironically, considering both his earlier stance on relocation of the Kamloops Indian Band and his support of the antituberculosis campaign, the Conservative candidate, former Kamloops mayor John Robinson, was one of the plan's opponents.

Following the election, the new Liberal MP T.G. McBride lobbied for the adoption of the scheme. Kamloops City Council and the business community (recently reorganized into the Kamloops Board of Trade) were on record in support of the proposal. In May 1922, the medical staff of the Royal Inland Hospital added their voice to the chorus. A petition to the DSCR noted the "most satisfactory" local climate, and stated that the proximity to transportation routes made the Kamloops Indian Reserve the ideal site for the proposed colony. The signatories of the petition were Kamloops' most prominent medical men: J.S. Burris, H.L. Burris, Houle, Irving, and Willoughby. Not until May 1922, when for practical and financial reasons the Board of Tuberculosis Consultants reported strongly against the whole idea of tuberculosis colonies, did the proposal fade from local attention. Denison himself, just before his move to eastern Canada, seems to have had the last word. In a lengthy article in *The Tranquillian*, he again set out in detail all the elements and benefits of the scheme. He urged that the Kamloops Indian Band be moved from its "undesirable proximity" to Kamloops to the Harper Ranch. The proposal received no further attention.[6]

Building, Expansion, Improvement

The provincial government set out to develop and expand the institution at Tranquille precisely as the British Columbia Anti-Tuberculosis Society had envisioned. While financial constraints were by no means eliminated, the Tranquille Sanatorium during most of the 1920s enjoyed both the moral and financial support of a government keen to make a success of the provincially-operated institution. Through the medical superintendent, senior staff at Tranquille had a direct link with the provincial secretary (the cabinet minister responsible for Tranquille) and with other institutions operated by the government, most notably the institution and farm at Essondale. Plans for the much-needed nurses' home were drawn up, and proposals to build new farm buildings and doctors' accommodations were being considered by the end of 1921.

One of the first principles of the Anti-Tuberculosis Society continued by the provincial government was that the sanatorium should be self-sufficient in its food supply. Self-sufficiency would also help to ensure the quality of the diet of patients—a crucial element in successful care of the tubercular. With only occasional exceptions due to unfavourable weather or crop and animal disease, the Alexandra Ranch, since its early years of operation, had managed to satisfy the food requirements of the institution. However, the opening of the Infirmary in 1919 had changed that. Capacity increased from 130 patients to 210, and would reach 230 once the problem of nurses' accommodation had been addressed. Clearly, if the Tranquille Sanatorium were to be self-sufficient in food once more, considerably more ranch land would be required.

The government's preferred solution to this problem was the same as that of the Anti-Tuberculosis Society. The adjacent Cooney ranch provided not only all the land that was necessary, but also had the considerable advantage of proximity. According to Strachan, the Cooney ranch buildings and the stock had deteriorated substantially since the death in 1917 of its founder Charles Cooney. The property remained highly desirable nevertheless, and, for the first time, the Cooney family indicated a willingness to sell. Therefore, the government approached Cooney's widow Elizabeth with an offer to purchase in the summer of 1922.

The events that followed created a legacy of bitterness in the Cooney family that remains to this day. Elizabeth Cooney and her son, Eugene, were offended by the government's offer of just over $47,000 for the 580-acre ranch, an offer that was to include all stock and lease land entitlements. The Cooney family claimed that much higher offers had been refused in the past and that the low offer was an insult to the memory of Charles Cooney. According to family memory, Cooney had magnanimously donated many acres of land to the Anti-Tuberculosis Society in 1912 when a survey error was discovered during the railway construction. After consideration, the Cooney family followed the advice of their Kamloops lawyer, Frederick Fulton, and refused to accept the government's offer.

It has been alleged that the government negotiators threatened expropriation and tried to bribe Eugene, who was an employee at the Alexandra Ranch. According to the Cooney family history published in the late 1970s, Eugene was promised a lifelong job if he could persuade his mother to agree to the sale. Much to the consternation of the Cooney family, Fulton changed his advice and began to urge acceptance of the government's offer. On condition that the family cemetery be maintained by the provincial government in perpetuity and that Elizabeth Cooney (over seventy years of age at the time of the agreement) could reside in the old ranch house until her death, Elizabeth and her son accepted the offer in November 1922.[7]

As Strachan went to work on the former Cooney property, so too did government construction crews get to work on the sanatorium itself, and, for a period of two years, the sound of construction was rarely absent from Tranquille. Within a year of the takeover, a spur line from the train station (after 1918, part of the Canadian National rail system) to the powerhouse was completed, as were new cement silos, a horse barn, a dairy barn and root cellars. Four staff cottages were built, and the long-awaited nurses' home, located just to the east of the Infirmary was officially opened by Governor General Viscount Byng in July 1922. Renovations and repairs to existing buildings took place throughout the following year, and in 1923, a new schoolhouse was constructed. The old cottages, built during the early days of the operation of the sanatorium and known as "the shacks," were replaced by five new cure cottages. These were located in front of the Main Building and were intended as accommodation for patients in the rehabilitative stages of treatment.

The new cottages were soon considered as a model for a scheme of housing in Kamloops intended for tubercular veterans. After the shelving of the scheme to locate a tuberculosis colony on the site of the Kamloops Indian Reserve, local MP T.G. McBride proposed that suitable housing should be built in Kamloops. The rental housing would allow veterans to remain for an extended period in the healthy environs of the dry belt, close to the treatment centre at Tranquille and a local community familiar with the limitations the disease placed upon its victims. The DSCR, noting both the unwillingness of Kamloops landlords to rent accommodation to tubercular veterans and the inability of pensioned and disabled veterans to purchase homes at market prices, placed $15,000 in the estimates of 1925 for the construction of five cottages at Kamloops. The scheme had the support of the Red Cross, the *Vancouver Province* and the *Victoria Times*, and the Tranquille branch of the influential Tuberculous Veterans' Association, which was the successor to the Invalided Tubercular Soldiers' Welfare League.

T.G. McBride visited Tranquille to examine the cure cottages and the residences occupied by staff. A committee that included Kamloops mayor S.C. Burton, Dr. Robert Irving, and others prominent in local affairs set to work on site selection and contract consideration. However, within six months and without any construction undertaken, the scheme was shelved. J.R. Pyper and the Tuberculous Veterans' Association at Tranquille became convinced that only a national scheme would suffice. They believed that the small scheme at Kamloops would only delay or prevent the DSCR from considering a grander proposal. Their change of heart effectively ended further consideration of the scheme, which was not subsequently revived.[8]

At Tranquille, water supply for drinking purposes and the treatment of sewage continued to present problems. Drinking water from the wells was described as "often muddy, unpalatable and not of the kind to help a patient quench his thirst."[9] The treatment of sewage was also of serious concern. A new sewage system was put in place in 1924, but it too proved unsatisfactory. The system was extended in 1927 to take the sewage even further away from the institutional buildings. The sewage was discharged into Kamloops Lake in front of the low lying fields used as horse meadows by the sanatorium ranch. The discharge occurred uncomfortably near the ranch house still inhabited by Elizabeth Cooney.

After May 1927, water for sanatorium purposes was also drawn from the same pool used for irrigation purposes just above the lower dam a mile up the creek. The wells were abandoned and everyone was pleased with the improved taste of the water from the new filtered gravity system. Heavy red sand from Wisconsin provided the filtration, and the supply of water was described as "inexhaustible." New hydrants were installed throughout the grounds, and the ninety-pound water pressure provided the institution for the first time with adequate fire protection. However, each year during the spring, drinking water had to be boiled to avoid the threat of contamination from the remaining prospectors who still lived along Tranquille Creek north of the sanatorium. The laboratory tested the water quality constantly, only rarely expressing concern at the results, but noting the turbidity during the spring run-off. It would be another ten years before the water supply of the sanatorium would receive further attention.

Life at the San

Everyday life at a sanatorium for patients and staff is difficult to describe, especially to those who have never visited or been confined to an institution. Official reports, from either a private organization or a government department, reveal little of the human aspects of hospital care and often seem to go to great lengths to conceal more than they illuminate. This was unfortunately the case at Tranquille until the end of the war years. However, the soldier-patients managed to change that—though not completely, not permanently, and not even intentionally—after 1918. Some of the new patients possessed skills that they sought to put to good use while they resided at Tranquille. Two photographers, along with a small group of newspaper men and aspiring writers, combined to leave a written and photographic legacy that makes the decade of the 1920s the most accessible of all the years the sanatorium was open.

The Tranquillian, though containing less local news and taking on a more official tone, continued to provide insight into the day-to-day life at the sanatorium. The photographic work of George Lothian presents a visual record through the post-war years until the mid-1920s. Lothian came to Tranquille as a patient towards the end of the war. An avid photographer, he produced postcard views of the sanatorium that were sold to raise funds for library purchases. Building upon his photographer's skills, he was appointed as the institution's first x-ray technician. His photographs provide an excellent visual record of the changes at the sanatorium. Many of his views are included in *The Tranquillian* and in the annual reports issued by the government during the early 1920s. Another patient particularly skilled with a camera, D. Lake Denman, first came to the sanatorium when the Balfour Sanatorium was closed in December 1920. Denman was a professional photographer who suffered from a mild but recurrent form of tuberculosis. Throughout the decade, he divided his time between work in Vancouver and recuperation at Tranquille, where he became a well-known and popular figure. Many of his images appear in the government's annual reports and *The Tranquillian*, especially later in the decade. His death in 1931 was much lamented at Tranquille, occurring ironically in the same year that George Lothian was dismissed due to cutbacks required by the economic depression. After his death, the rights to Lake Denman's photographs were acquired by the Camera Company of Vancouver. As hand-coloured postcards, they represented the most popular visual images of Tranquille until well after World War II.

As the photographs of Denman and Lothian and the columns of *The Tranquillian* indicate, daily life at the sanatorium seemed little affected by all the political wrangling and the administrative concerns. For the bed patients, hours of inactivity or boredom were relieved only by an occasional visitor, a book from the sanatorium library, a craft activity, or a programme on the radio headset. For ambulant patients, seasonal walks around the grounds and meal time in the dining room could add some additional interest to daily routines. For all patients, the early afternoon hours were a period of required inactivity: "the cure" was strictly enforced between 1 p.m. and 3 p.m. Sleeping on the porches was still very much part of the night time routine, though patients could now decide for themselves when the weather was too cold.

For everyone, including staff, the visits of individuals and groups provided a most welcome relief from daily patterns. The community of Kamloops was the source of most of these visitors during the inter-war years, just as it had been before the government takeover. The local Red Cross took over the philanthropic work of the Kamloops chapter of the Anti-Tuberculosis Society after 1921, and their regular visits (along with the magazines, cigarettes and clothing they brought) were welcomed, particularly by the poorer patients. It is interesting to note that, while smoking was frowned upon by the medical staff and condemned by articles in *The Tranquillian*, it was not actively prohibited at the sanatorium. The consumption of alcohol, on the other hand, was still strictly forbidden.

Of benefit to all were the frequent visits of local performing groups, which occurred particularly on seasonal occasions. The churches and service clubs also played a significant role, taking patients on drives and picnics, or sponsoring events and performances at the institution. The support provided by the organizations of Kamloops was so significant that any attempt to name here some of the contributors would only do a disservice to those unacknowledged. It was a rare group indeed that somehow failed to consider how their activity might be of benefit to the patients at the sanatorium. Visits by more famous organizations from out of the local area were also frequent. The Kitsilano High School Boys' Band, for example, was a regular visitor during the 1930s as it performed at Tranquille *en route* to or from national competitions and European tours.[10]

The Tranquillian itself provided a source of diversion as well. Though most of its columns were filled with didactic articles about the causes and treatment of tuberculosis, others offered literary criticism, history lessons, and humour. "The Knights of the Burning Brow" column told of the lives of famous victims of the disease. Keats, Mozart, Voltaire, Francis of Assisi and others were shown as examples that the disease could not crush the human spirit. In "The New Disease-Rhymatism," one writer spoke of the near mania in the 1920s at Tranquille amongst patients and staff for writing poetry. The sanatorium's poets were all hopeful of seeing their verses printed in *The Tranquillian*. Perhaps the most popular regular column was a literate satire of *The Diary of Samuel Pepys*. Writing as Peter Peeps, the author cryptically discusses the characters, foibles, and liaisons of Tranquille residents. "Peter Peeps' Diary" ran for many years, its author and allusions familiar to contemporary residents of Tranquille. Readers were also amused by frequent reference to Tranquille as "Bugtown," and to the "annual conventions" the mosquitoes held at the sanatorium. Perhaps many purchased the "Bugtite" cupholder, developed by a patient who regularly advertised her creation in *The Tranquillian* during the 1930s.

Patients did not depend entirely on visits and newspapers for their diversion. Many created their own activities. Annual elections for a mayor of Tranquille and a queen took place. Both occasions were parodies of elections elsewhere, sometimes raising funds for the Amusement Committee in the process, and providing diversion even for bed patients. Patient John Bruce Magee was re-elected annually as mayor throughout the 1920s. The two big annual festivities were Christmas and Hallowe'en. The auditorium in the Main Building was used annually to wait for the arrival of Santa's sleigh, and gifts were distributed to children, patients, and staff. At Hallowe'en, ambulant patients and staff in costume toured through all the buildings. Though Dr. Lapp attempted to limit the procession to certain buildings after 1929, the Hallowe'en tradition survived for many years.

Motion pictures and radio programmes were popular. Silent movies were shown in the hall of the Main Building in the 1920s using a projector purchased with funds donated from the Canteen, but silent movies became almost impossible to acquire after 1931. Tranquille's first talking-picture machine was purchased, also with Canteen funds, and on 30 November 1932 the Marx Brothers' *Monkey Business* became the first "talkie" shown at Tranquille. Weekly Wednesday showings were reserved for staff, while Thursday screenings were for patients only. On movie nights, the hall was called the Rex Theatre. Radio programme decisions were made by a vote of patients, and during the late 1930s, "Hockey Night in Canada" was always the popular choice on Saturday night.

Sports that required exertion were forbidden to patients. Consequently, no patients were involved in the soccer team that was formed in the early 1930s. The team had only a small population to draw from, but managed to win the Province Cup (donated by the *Vancouver Province*) three years in a row from 1932 to 1934 and, therefore, was entitled to keep the prize. The tennis club, headed by Mrs. Lapp, was for staff only, as was recreational horse riding. Swimming in Kamloops Lake was not permitted for staff or patients due to health concerns about the sewage disposal. Croquet on the lawns and, when the river was low, use of the small golf course in the late summer and fall were available to active patients. A small three-par putting green, located just behind the Main Building, was also popular.

The sports events that involved most patients, though only as spectators or organizers, were the Tranquille Races. The first Tranquille Turf Day was held on 14 May 1921 at the Tranquille

Meadows on the Alexandra Ranch. Ranch Superintendent Strachan was clerk of the course and prizes were offered for the cowboy race, the Indian race, a children's race, and a free-for-all race. The event was well attended and showed enough profit for the patients' Amusement Committee that a fall event was also planned for 1921. Both the spring and fall occasions became annual events. The highlights for many were apparently the Indian races. The Rocky Mountain Ranger Band played annually and, after 1923, the A.D. Lapp Cup was awarded to the winner of the Tranquille Half-Mile race. In 1924, five hundred people from Kamloops arrived aboard a train put on by the CNR especially for the event. As many as a thousand people attended until similar events in Kamloops started to reduce the crowds at Tranquille after 1926. The final Tranquille Turf Day was held in the spring of 1927.

Of course, not all aspects of life at Tranquille were so pleasant. A roach infestation in 1927 required the attention of a specialist from Seattle. A toxic powder was blown into cracks and crevices, and according to Lapp, "millions of these pests crawled out of their hiding places and died." The same specialist was called upon to deal with a bedbug problem in 1928.[11] However, the most persistent problem was with mosquitoes. Though references to the mosquito problem are absent from the records of the Anti-Tuberculosis Society, the Tranquille district seems to have bred a distinctly troublesome variety. The first superintendent, Dr. Irving, continued to speak of mosquitoes years after he had resigned, suggesting the insects had certainly been part of his experience. In early July 1921, the British Columbia Hospitals Association held its fourth annual convention in Kamloops and, one evening, delegates visited Tranquille. *The Tranquillian* reported that, after supper, the visitors "boarded their waiting motor cars and quickly passed out of the mosquito zone." A humorous article from a former patient suggested that somehow mosquitoes born and bred at Tranquille were immune to tuberculosis:

> Those [mosquitos] who are natives of Tranquille, and I believe that the majority of the mosquitos of B.C. live near the Sanatorium, feed with avidity...on the fluid extracts of T.B. patients, yet I have never yet met one that suffered from a cough, night sweats, or any of the recognized symptoms.[12]

Other references to mosquitoes preventing outdoor activities are frequent, and advertisements appeared regularly in *The Tranquillian* for Minard's Liniment, a product that promised to take the itch out of mosquito bites. One former resident recalls her mother wearing a beekeeper's outfit as protection against mosquitoes while she worked in her garden. Fragmentary evidence in government records indicates that from 1929 to 1936, when finances permitted, the Tranquille Sanatorium cooperated with Kamloops and North Kamloops in oiling wetland areas. When no money was available, as in 1933, the mosquito problem was severe.[13]

The Tranquille Tuberculosis Publicity Society

The Tranquillian, from its inception, served two purposes formerly addressed by the auxiliary branches of the Anti-Tuberculosis Society: publicity and fundraising. First the society and then the government saw the newspaper as a way of educating the public and those who suffered from the disease about the issues surrounding tuberculosis care and prevention. Articles by medical personnel in British Columbia and from across Canada discussed history and treatment in every issue. Expected initially to be self-supporting, the "sanmag" quickly became a profitable venture through subscriptions and advertising revenues. Subscriptions were taken out by other sanatoria, by branches of the ITSWL, by interested doctors and family members of those at the sanatorium. At the time of the government takeover, approximately three-quarters of the more than 1,000 copies printed were being sent outside Tranquille. Throughout the remainder of the decade, the paper would have a circulation of between 1,500 and 2,000 copies. Most advertisers were from Kamloops or Vancouver, and all advertisers seem to have been welcomed. Advertisements to purchase a strong Rainier beer must have seemed incongruous to sanatorium residents who were expressly forbidden to drink alcohol while at the sanatorium. Nevertheless, the income generated by the newspaper allowed it to expand quickly to ten pages by August 1920 and to twenty pages by June 1922.

At a general meeting of patients in January 1921, it was decided to have a four-member board made responsible for the production of *The Tranquillian*. The medical superintendent would work with three patient representatives of the ITSWL, the Amusement Committee, and the Civilian Comforts Committee. The arrangement became more formal late in 1922. At the suggestion of Dr. Lapp, the Tranquille Tuberculosis Publicity Society was created and registered under the *British Columbia Societies Act* to oversee the production of the newspaper and to administer the profits. The editor and a staff of three patients were to be paid. However, patient involvement was reduced by the reorganization as the new ten-member board was dominated by doctors and senior employees at Tranquille. The content was also to be more strictly supervised by Superintendent Lapp. After a series of editors and a short-lived move of production to the Rotary Clinic in Vancouver, former patient and veteran J.R. Pyper of Kamloops became editor in 1922. Though he would successfully edit "the sanmag" until 1936, and though columns about life at Tranquille continued to be featured regularly, *The Tranquillian* became a less lively publication with a more official tone. Tranquille patients began to complain in the early 1920s that there was not enough news of the sanatorium.

The Tranquille Tuberculosis Publicity Society typically managed to generate a small annual profit after paying sales commissions, printing costs and the salaries of Pyper and his production staff. Revenues were derived primarily from advertising and subscriptions, though donations from the public were again solicited. It is significant that, in most years, apart from a grant to the society of $100 per month from the provincial government, hardly any donations were received. Following his appointment as travelling provincial medical health officer in 1923, former Tranquille doctor A.S. Lamb commented on the financial burden placed on the provincial government. He saw the public's disinterest as a consequence of the government takeover. He wrote:

> The inevitable result followed. Whenever a government takes over anything, the people lose interest...All these voluntary organizations lapsed and with them all the propaganda that they had been carrying on, ceased also.[14]

Surprisingly, for one so familiar with the circumstances of the Anti-Tuberculosis Society, Dr. Lamb was confusing cause and effect in his assessment. If donation of time or resources is a measure of public interest, the public had lost interest well before the government takeover. With the exception of the still active New Westminster chapter, the auxiliary societies had ceased to exist in all but name by Christmas 1921. Their dissemination of propaganda and their fundraising had diminished sharply even before the war brought a focus upon soldier-related charity, and had all but ceased prior to the government takeover. Sympathy for veterans brought a revival in charitable contributions for a time after the war. The most durable examples of this renewed charitable involvement came from the Kamloops chapters of the Imperial Order of the Daughters of the Empire (IODE) and the Red Cross. In 1920, the IODE chapter donated a pleasure launch (named "Stobart" in honour of its donors) and a pool table, and the Kamloops Red Cross for many years maintained its programme of regular visits to the sanatorium and contributions to indigent patients. But the reluctance of the public to contribute to the Tranquille Tuberculosis Publicity Society during the 1920s continued. This was a continuation of pre-war and wartime patterns, not simply a consequence of government intervention.

The society's profits from sales of *The Tranquillian* were always expended in the interests of Tranquille patients. The sanatorium's first radio, complete with headsets for every bed patient, was purchased by the society in 1925. Books for the patient library and clothing and toiletries for poorer patients were paid for with profits from *The Tranquillian*. In 1926, the sale of Christmas seals was initiated with considerable success. Nearly 200,000 were sold province-wide, bringing the society nearly $400 in profit. The Tranquille seal campaign was repeated in 1927. As part of a reorganization in 1927, the society shortened its name to the Tranquille Tuberculosis Society and agreed to become part of the national campaign to sell the Canadian Tuberculosis Association's seals. Typically, in subsequent years, a "folding bee" was held in October at the nurses' home to prepare the seals for distribution.

Even during the Depression years, though sales of Christmas seals fell sharply, the Tranquille Tuberculosis Society was able to continue its antituberculosis work. The profit from Christmas seals purchased a portable x-ray machine and paid the wages of a travelling clinic nurse. Josephine Peters, working from Kamloops and travelling throughout the Interior, held that position for many years. However, reduced revenues from advertising after 1929 challenged the ability of *The Tranquillian* to remain profitable. By 1932, despite a monthly circulation of between 2,300 and 2,400 copies, the newspaper was no longer self-supporting.[15] Fortunately for poorer patients at Tranquille, the profits from the operation of the Canteen after 1929 were sufficient to replace the loss of contributions from *The Tranquillian*.

Continuing Patterns and Problems

In other ways too, the situation under government administration remained the same as that encountered by the Anti-Tuberculosis Society. The patient population was still largely made up of males of working age, and the number of non-paying patients continued to grow. Drawn for the most part from the working population of the province—miners, loggers, labourers—the male patients were often in no position to pay weekly fees. As the income derived from the DSCR diminished with the steadily decreasing numbers of soldier patients, more room existed for civilian cases. Typically, the new admissions were unable to pay the required fees, leaving municipalities and the provincial government responsible for their maintenance. The per diem contribution from municipal governments was raised to $2.50 in 1921, but ultimately the money was coming from the same source: taxpayers. The operating deficit in the first year of government operation stood at just over $90,000. It rose in the second year to over $130,000, as the number of indigent patients increased to more than a third of the total patient population.[16] By 1935, with only five percent of patients paying their own fees, the institution was almost completely dependent upon the government for payment of fees.

During its years of operation, the British Columbia Anti-Tuberculosis Society stated regularly that the preponderance of advanced cases prevented beds from being available to those who had a greater chance of being cured. In his first annual report as medical superintendent, Dr. Lapp echoed that concern. Lapp noted that some patients had occupied beds for years but could not be discharged, and urged that a separate facility be constructed in order that Tranquille could cure, rather than just care for, tubercular patients.

However, just two years later, he was arguing that the care of advanced cases at Tranquille was part of the institution's mandate. He noted it was well worth treating even the far advanced to alleviate their suffering and to prevent the spread of infection that would result by denying them admission. With no plans for construction of a separate facility, it was clearly necessary to continue to treat all cases at Tranquille regardless of seriousness. Political realities no doubt suggested it was just as necessary for the new medical superintendent to submit reports free from implied criticism of the government responsible for running the institution. Though figures changed daily, advanced and far-advanced patients generally occupied two-thirds of the beds at Tranquille throughout the 1920s and 1930s. Death rates were high amongst this group. The grim reality is that Tranquille typically would see one death per week and, perhaps, from amongst the despondent, one suicide each year.

One other aspect of sanatorium operation that did not change under government operation was the high turnover of staff. The difficulties of retaining capable nurses and support staff at a time of inflationary wage pressures was a source of great discouragement to the Anti-Tuberculosis Society after World War I. Wage pressures stabilized for most of the 1920s, and wage reductions and unemployment generally prevailed during the 1930s, but Tranquille suffered continuously from an inability to retain employees. Retaining a full complement of nurses was particularly difficult. Between April 1928 and April 1929, for example, twenty-four nurses left the institution. Some left for other positions; a few left to get married, but many cited the isolation, the crowded living conditions of the nurses' home, and the poor working conditions as their reasons for resigning.[17]

Poor living quarters were the main impediment to retaining support staff during this period as well. As employees of the sanatorium, they were required to live at Tranquille, but accommodation for them was completely inadequate. Construction of the farm boarding house in 1925, the maids' home in 1926, and the men's boarding house during 1927-28 addressed the problem, but never managed to eliminate it. When the opening of the Greaves Building further increased the capacity of the sanatorium, additions to the nurses' home and the men's boarding house were required in 1929. A survey of all employees in 1931 revealed that of 168 sanatorium employees,

114 had been appointed since 1928; of nineteen ranch staff, none had been employed there before 1928.[18] Concerns were regularly expressed by Dr. Lapp about the quality of the staff the institution was able to attract under such conditions of instability.

Retaining senior medical and non-medical staff was not as much of a problem. Though accommodation for them was not ideal, it was far superior to that of the nurses, maids, and male support staff. Four detached staff residences were built in 1923, and others were added in 1926. However, even the senior staff had to wait until the end of the decade before the government voted funds for appropriate housing. Five detached residences, an apartment building for single doctors, and a fine new home for the medical superintendent were all constructed along the road leading to the Tranquille station in 1928-29. Assistant physicians generally stayed at Tranquille for several years, as did the matron. Miss M. Hodgetts, a Tranquille nurse who had been promoted to matron in 1923 when J.A. Morrice left the institution, resigned for health reasons in 1926. She was replaced by Blanche Bibby, another former Tranquille nurse with wartime experience in France. Bibby left her position at a sanatorium in California in order to return to Tranquille and would remain as matron for ten years.

Decades after Koch's discovery of 1882, a cure for tuberculosis seemed as distant as ever. Except in a few significant respects, the care patients received at Tranquille during the inter-war years was remarkably similar to that supervised by Irving, Vrooman, and Houle. Early experiments with graduated work therapy were not continued, though occupational therapy and carefully monitored exercise were encouraged. Eggs were no longer the staple diet, but rest, good food and exposure to fresh air and sunshine remained essential requirements of treatment. Nevertheless, the institution was not slow to incorporate medical and technological advances in its operation. X-ray capabilities were added in 1916, and by the early 1920s all patients, employees, and their families were x-rayed regularly. A laboratory was added in 1923 to provide further diagnostic tools for medical treatment. Applying another of Koch's discoveries—that guinea pigs had no resistance whatsoever to tuberculosis—the laboratory used thousands of the creatures over the years for diagnostic and research purposes. Both x-ray and laboratory facilities were upgraded frequently as the years went by.

Surgical treatment was also available to selected Tranquille patients. Though small operating rooms were included in the Infirmary, Tranquille did not possess a major operating theatre. Nor did it have trained surgeons on its medical staff. Dr. Irving and especially Dr. J.S. Burris acted as consulting surgeons after 1919, performing all but minor procedures at the Royal Inland Hospital in Kamloops. Lung collapse surgery for sanatorium patients was performed as early as 1922. The surgical requirements of modern treatment of tuberculosis increased steadily with each passing year, and by the early 1930s, it was apparent that Tranquille required its own surgical unit. In 1934, Lapp and assistant superintendent Chisholm visited sanatoria throughout Canada and the United States to study surgical arrangements. However, plans to include funds in the provincial estimates for a comprehensive surgery at Tranquille were shelved due to the continuing financial restraint caused by the economic depression. In 1935, Dr. J.S. Burris at the Royal Inland Hospital performed the first pneumolysis operation in western Canada, underscoring the need for a facility at Tranquille. It was not until November 1936 that Lapp was finally able to announce government approval for Tranquille to acquire its own surgical unit.[19]

Provincial Politics, Local Politics

The Tranquille Sanatorium was accustomed to political controversy. Prior to Denison's proposal, political issues had attended the founding of the sanatorium, the appointment and dismissal of superintendents, the operations of the British Columbia Anti-Tuberculosis Society, the soldier complaints, and the propriety of both federal and provincial government intervention. After 1921, partisan provincial politics could be added to the list. Building contracts, for example, were closely scrutinized. The limited accommodation for nurses available in the Administration Building was completely inadequate, and had been since the opening of the Infirmary Building in 1919. A separate building for the matron and nearly two dozen nurses was, therefore, one of the first priorities of the government at Tranquille. The politically Conservative *Kamloops Standard-Sentinel* demanded to know why the Liberal government had awarded the contract for the construction of the nurses' home in 1922 to an out-of-province firm, while lower bids from Kamloops-area firms were rejected. In contrast, newspapers favouring the Liberal government, such as the *Kamloops Telegram*, the *Victoria Daily Times*, and the *Vancouver Sun*, extolled the virtues of a "superbly-run institution" at Tranquille throughout the decade of the 1920s. Though medical appointments seem to have been generally spared from controversies, all other senior staff soon found their terms of employment subject to partisan debate. Relatively soon after the government took responsibility for the institution, it became a common assumption, especially in Kamloops and in Conservative circles, that those employed at Tranquille must necessarily be Liberal supporters.

The government had always to contend with the criticism that it was not doing enough. The Tranquille Sanatorium had never been able to eliminate waiting lists, and with an expanding provincial economy attracting a growing population, pressure on the institution increased during the 1920s. Consequently, in 1927, the government announced plans to use the Greaves legacy to assist in the construction of a 100-bed expansion at Tranquille.

The announcement attracted attention from Ottawa. The federal government saw the opportunity to address the high tuberculosis rate among British Columbia's Native population. As wards of the federal government, the Native people of British Columbia were ineligible for admittance to provincially-run institutions unless they were veterans. Though it had long been recognized that the rate of infection amongst Natives was at least ten times greater than that among the European population, there were no facilities or treatment programmes whatsoever for Native people.

Finally deciding at least to investigate, the federal government appointed University of British Columbia professor Dr. H.W. Hill, Dr. Vrooman and Dr. Lamb to conduct an extensive survey of the problem. Their report led the federal government to initiate discussions with the provincial government about the possibility of a jointly funded facility at Tranquille. They proposed that a 200-bed facility be constructed, with 100 beds being set aside for Native patients. The arrangement would have been similar to that involving the soldier-patients that had led to construction of the Infirmary in 1919. However, the two levels of government could not agree on terms, and, by the summer of 1927, negotiations were abandoned. Though a ward at Vancouver General Hospital was made available for Native sufferers of tuberculosis in 1939, it would not be until 1941 that a separate facility for Natives was opened by the Indian Affairs Branch at Coqualeetza, near Sardis. Until after World War II, only Natives who were veterans were eligible for admission to Tranquille. Like all other buildings at Tranquille, the new building was to care for British Columbia's non-Native and non-Asian tubercular population.

The new building was clearly intended by the Liberal government to be the showpiece of the institution and of the government's provincial health care policies. Premier John Oliver visited Tranquille twice in 1926 to discuss the project with Dr. Lapp, and $250,000 was included in the estimates for construction in early 1927. The provincial government called for tenders in September 1927 for the construction of a 100-bed facility at Tranquille. Included in the building programme would be a new home for the medical superintendent, a small block of apartments for other senior medical staff, a large boarding house for male help, underground tunnels to link the new structure with the Infirmary and the Main Building, and an addition to the nurses' home. Funds accumulated through the Greaves bequest were earmarked for the building project. By the time construction was completed more than a year later, close to $400,000 had been spent, nearly three-quarters of this from the Greaves legacy.

Again, during the summer and fall of 1928, the sanatorium was alive with the noise of construction. However, the Liberal administration would not survive to see the task completed, as Simon Tolmie's Conservatives won the summer election of 1928. Suspecting that the sanatorium was a nest of Liberals, Tolmie did not view the institution with as much favour as had his predecessor. After a visit in November, he and Provincial Secretary S.L. Howe declared the sanatorium to be "one of the finest institutions on the North American continent." However, there was an implication in the complimentary description that extravagant expenditure had made it so. When the Greaves Building was completed in January, both Tolmie and Howe advised Lapp they found it impossible to leave Victoria due to government business. Patients began to move to the lower two floors. Only after accepting an invitation to the Kamloops Bull Show did

Tolmie manage to find time to open the new building officially. He advised Lapp on 25 March 1929 that he would do so two days later.

Even with such short notice, the event attracted 150 people on the afternoon of 27 March. Accompanied by Howe and the minister of education, Tolmie paid particular tribute to J.B. Greaves, whose bequest to the British Columbia Anti-Tuberculosis Society ten years earlier had made the construction possible and in whose honour the building was named. A modern three-storey concrete structure, served by an elevator, and finished in white stucco with a red tiled roof, the Greaves Building was certainly an impressive sight. The patients' rooms were of various sizes, and though there were no verandahs, folding windows permitted each room to be quickly converted to an open-air porch. On the upper floor was a solarium with violet-ray glass to allow patients to enjoy the benefits of sunshine and a view of the Thompson valley. A concrete tunnel, heated and lit by electricity, connected the new structure to the Service Building, the Main Building, and the Laundry to facilitate the movement of goods, food, and people, especially during winter. Taking the key from its purple velvet cushion and inserting it in the lock, Premier Tolmie declared the building officially opened.

With the opening of the Greaves Building, the number of beds available in British Columbia to treat tuberculosis rose to 400. All were at Tranquille, except approximately eighty beds available at Vancouver General Hospital. Patients were immediately transferred to Tranquille from the overcrowded ward at VGH. Within a year, Lapp reported that all beds in the new building were occupied, but the waiting list had not been eliminated. More than one hundred victims of tuberculosis waited for vacancies to permit their admission to Tranquille. The opening of the Greaves Building highlighted a long-standing problem at the institution: at least thirty full-time nurses were required at the sanatorium after 1929.

The Conservative Party was in office only a few months before Provincial Secretary Howe ordered an investigation of operations at the politically suspect sanatorium. The Conservatives had won a narrow majority in the Kamloops riding, but the vote at Tranquille favoured the Liberal candidate by a margin of more than two to one. The report received by Howe concluded that, though the medical work was "admirable in its character," the performance of Lapp's senior non-medical assistants and the ranch management was deficient. Most of the deficiencies were found in known Liberal supporters. Amongst others, ranch superintendent David Strachan was dismissed as was long-time bursar and former patient Alexander Whitecross.

Strachan had been so long in charge that he was himself practically an institution by 1929. Active in local agricultural organizations, he received much attention throughout the 1920s as the dairy herd at Tranquille set national milk production records. Pedigreed Holsteins Alexandra Verona May and Alexandra Orne Mack shared the fame.[20] But his political inclinations negated his achievements in the eyes of the new administration, which also took the opportunity to redefine the position. The man in charge of the ranch was to be known henceforth as the farm manager. He would possess less autonomy than his predecessors, as the farm was placed more directly under the control of the medical superintendent.

Sixty years of age, new farm manager William Jackson once had worked as a farm hand for William Fortune. The operation he took over was expected to provide the food requirements of approximately 600 people. However, the administration of the ranch had become simpler in two respects. The sheep had been sold in 1926 when the flock, which had long interfered with the cattle herd, was plagued with poisonous weed problems. Just a year later, the poultry operation, which had been expanded by Strachan to include turkey raising, was ended due to health concerns. Apart from fruits and vegetables, Jackson was free therefore to focus upon swine, beef, and dairy cattle. He did not apparently repeat Strachan's successful 1928 attempt at growing tobacco.

Jackson strove to maintain all aspects of the agricultural operation, but his heart seems to have been with the beef operation, which he hoped to see increase to one thousand head. Dr. Lapp was impressed by the new management style of Jackson and looked forward to seeing the farm again provide all the beef requirements of the sanatorium. That goal was reached in 1933. Lapp advised the provincial secretary that not only had the sanatorium sent its first shipment of beef to Essondale, it also hoped to supply the Provincial Home in Kamloops that year with all its beef requirements.[21] Lapp spoke especially highly of the improvements Jackson made to the appearance of the ranch buildings, noting that by 1932, the whole farm had a well-kept appearance "quite the opposite of that of a year or two ago."

The *Kamloops Sentinel* agreed. It reported favourably upon Jackson's sixteen miles of whitewashed fencing all "as straight as a string," the newly-planted orchards, the successful introduction of bees, and the operation of an abattoir that could handle 550 carcasses a year with "a complete absence of any vexatious odour."[22] The heavy operating loss shown by the ranch in Jackson's first year of stewardship was attributed by the annual report to the need to reduce Strachan's excessively high valuation of livestock. Lapp stated that difficulties in running the farm consistently at a profit after 1930 were due to depressed prices throughout the Kamloops district.

The new Conservative administration in Victoria expressed concern about two other matters: employment practices and the operation of a private business on sanatorium property. The policy of employing former patients whenever possible had been followed by both the British Columbia Anti-Tuberculosis Society and the provincial government. Jobs ranged from a few hours per week as part of a rehabilitation programme to full employment. Considering the constant difficulties in acquiring competent staff, the policy was as much a matter of necessity for the employer as it was a kindness towards people whose ability to work at full time employment had been compromised by tuberculosis. The former patients were concentrated in the jobs requiring less physical exertion, being employed primarily in office and clerical positions in administration or in preparation of *The Tranquillian*. Alexander Whitecross, for example, had studied accountancy for years while a patient at Tranquille through correspondence courses before becoming the institution's business agent in 1919. George Lothian's experience as a photographer made him a logical choice for x-ray technician when the sanatorium acquired that technology. The new government was concerned that twenty-eight of the 168 people employed by the institution in 1929 were former patients, suspicious that their employment was due more to Liberal connections than to abilities. They threatened to discontinue the policy and to dismiss all former patients from employment, but, after dismissing known-Liberal

Alexander Whitecross, were content to permit the practice to continue.[23]

The operation of a privately owned general store also concerned the new administration. Operated for many years by J.M. Cropley, the store offered for sale to staff and patients basic groceries as well as candy, cigarettes, and ice cream. The government denied Cropley the right to continue and forced him to accept its offer for the current stock, an offer based on personal notes from both Dr. Lapp and the new bursar, Mr. Jefferis. Notices went up at the store in the summer of 1929 that the business (to be known henceforth as the Canteen) was to be run for the benefit of the institution and not for private profit. The loans from Lapp and Jefferis were quickly repaid and the Canteen would generate funds for the general purposes of the sanatorium for the next thirty years. Complaints from Kamloops merchants in the 1930s that the Canteen was "encroaching upon their business" indicate that monthly sales were significant. Most of the sales were generated by cigarettes, candy, soft drinks and cosmetics, but shoes and clothing were also available.[24]

Political considerations notwithstanding, by the late 1920s the sanatorium at Tranquille had become one of the premier tourist attractions in the Kamloops district. The *Sentinel* editorialized in 1927 that the sanatorium was the city's "beauty spot, a 'sight' to show strangers, something to be proud of."[25] No longer was a visit to the Tranquille Sanatorium simply a matter of public duty, philanthropy, or medical concern. Automobiles and road improvements made the location more readily accessible, and the view from the institution up and down Kamloops Lake was magnificent. However, the feature that drew most sightseers to Tranquille was the gardens. Largely neglected during the early years of operation due to financial constraints, landscaping at Tranquille began to receive attention during the war years, and, after 1921, the government made landscaping a priority. Especially around the four larger buildings—Main, East Pavilion, West Pavilion and the Infirmary—a variety of trees and shrubbery as well as perennial and seasonal flowers were planted. In front of the West Pavilion, an attempt was made to create a modified oriental garden with ponds, running water, an arched bridge and footpaths. This portion of the grounds was commonly referred to as the sunken garden. *The Tranquillian* commented:

> What was waste ground with nothing but weeds flourishing on it in front of the west pavilion is now a sunken garden and is, in the opinion of some visitors from Vancouver Island, the equal of anything to be seen in the famous Butchart Gardens.[26]

Imported wild pheasants and other birds, protected within the Tranquille Wildlife Preserve after 1926, added another visual pleasure for visitors. *The Tranquillian* boasted that the sanatorium was "unquestionably the showplace of Kamloops." The approval in Kamloops of Jackson's fencing project had a great deal to do with the knowledge that the appearance of a tourist attraction was being enhanced. The grounds received another attraction in 1934 when a huge granite stone basin was discovered southwest of Kamloops. Its historical significance as a Native artifact was quickly recognized, but because of its weight it was judged too expensive to move to the Provincial Museum in Victoria. It was hauled to Tranquille instead and located on the lawn behind the Main Building.[27] On fine summer days, only the awareness that the grounds were those of a tuberculosis hospital allowed the administration to keep the influx of visitors within manageable proportions.

The proliferation of private sanatoria in Kamloops, predicted by the early opponents of the Tranquille facility, had not occurred. Dr. Irving operated his private sanatorium, first as the Riverside Cottage Sanatorium until 1914, and then as the Sunny View Sanatorium in the Powers Addition southwest of the city centre. At both locations he was assisted by Gertrude Blackford, who had been employed as a nurse at Tranquille as early as 1909. However, perhaps because of a dearth of patients able to afford the $60 monthly fees, Irving's sanatorium was no longer in business by the early 1920s. A smaller operation was then opened in the downtown area and run until the early 1930s by Mrs. James Whitmore, who for a time had been a nurse's aide at Tranquille. Despite the fears of the 1900s and despite the post-war promotion of the city's beneficial climate, the region had not become a magnet for the nation's tubercular population.

Though fears of contamination had all but disappeared and though the economic advantages of the Tranquille Sanatorium were apparent, there remained amongst some in Kamloops an attitude that can only be described as mean-spirited. The allegations of political favouritism at Tranquille were frequent enough to be commonplace, and complaints about mismanagement from dismissed employees were perhaps also to be expected. However, the sanatorium was rarely free from petty local allegations of inappropriate behaviour or indefensible policies. A police investigation in 1931 sought to discover the source of anonymous letters to MLAs criticizing the sanatorium on various points. Letters in the *Kamloops Sentinel* in 1932 drew a rare public response from Dr. Lapp, who felt the critical atmosphere keenly. He once advised the provincial secretary's office: "I go to Kamloops only when necessary and stay there only as long as is necessary as I always feel that the village-minded inhabitants of that town criticize whenever they see me in there."[28]

If Dr. Lapp welcomed an isolated existence at Tranquille, the institution could not escape the ravages of time and economic forces. The attractive buildings needed regular cosmetic attention, but money was not always available for paint and improvements. Though Lapp noted in 1934 that the buildings had never looked worse during his twelve years at the institution, his request for paint was denied. The flagpole, erected with such pride by the British Columbia Anti-Tuberculosis Society in front of the administration building in 1912, presented a danger and was removed in 1934 because of its rotting base. The economic situation of the 1930s seriously affected the operation of Tranquille. In 1931, the prospect of staff cuts and wage reductions had to be faced. Though costs of goods were being reduced, government revenues were shrinking even more rapidly. In November 1931, Dr. Lapp received an order from the provincial secretary to reduce staff. Seven people, including x-ray technician George Lothian were dismissed to achieve a saving of more than $10,000 on a payroll that had exceeded $150,000 annually. Lapp noted that those remaining "shouldered the extra burden good-naturedly" and that patients had not felt any change. Staff may have found it difficult to remain good-natured in 1933 when a round of salary cuts occurred for the remaining 180 employees. Those earning under $1,225 annually saw their incomes reduced by three percent, while those earning more than that amount suffered cuts of between five and seventeen percent.[29]

The return to power of the Liberals in 1933 brought another round of investigations and staff changes. Citing persistent criticism from Kamloops of the Tranquille operation, the new provincial secretary, George Weir, appointed a departmental commission of enquiry. Victoria lawyer C.H. O'Halloran, Vancouver General Hospital superintendent Dr. A.K. Haywood and UBC animal husbandry professor Dr. H. King visited Tranquille and Kamloops in late February 1934 to hold public hearings and to interview staff. The public hearing at the courthouse in Kamloops on 27 February revealed the extent to which the official attitude of the city had changed over the years. Without exception, the commission heard praise from everyone, including the mayor, who noted that the sanatorium was "a great asset directly to Kamloops." No criticism of the administration at the institution was expressed.[30] Nevertheless, rumours given a wide circulation in Kamloops insisted that among the many heads about to roll would be included those of Dr. Lapp, farm manager Jackson and bursar Jefferis. With the exception of Lapp, the rumours were correct.

The political appointees of the Conservatives were found by the Liberals to be performing inadequately in their jobs. Premier Duff Pattullo announced in June that Jackson would be replaced. Jackson received the news just as he was completing the construction of a dam at the headwaters of Tranquille Creek, replacing Strachan's dam of fifteen years earlier. Three hundred and thirty feet long, the new dam was eighty feet wide at its base and, according to the *Kamloops Sentinel* would provide the grateful community of Tranquille with the best water in the world and excellent fire protection.[31] UBC professor R.L. Davis, with no previous managerial experience, became the fourth farm manager of the sanatorium a few days later, and by the end of the year his annual salary was raised by $300.

The commission declared the accounting methods of Jefferis were unacceptable (though no dishonesty was alleged) and recommended his replacement. Apparently with Lapp's support, Jefferis was able to resist the pressure to resign until December 1935, when he declined the offer of a position at Essondale and purchased the G.G. Foss general store at Barriere. The new appointee, E.M. Selkirk—married with three children—moved into the small bursar's house. The entire process was profoundly discouraging to Lapp. Less than a year later, for personal reasons, Matron Blanche Bibby also submitted her resignation, being replaced in an acting capacity by Miss Barter. With the exception of Dr. Lapp, the senior personnel at the institution—matron, farm manager, and bursar—were all new to their positions. And the medical superintendent was becoming restless in his.

End of an Era

Dr. Lapp's style of administration left the impression with many that he was aloof and disinterested in the lives of the people he worked with. *The Tranquillian* refers to him as being quiet, but does not comment otherwise upon his character. He does not seem to have been involved in clubs or activities at Tranquille or in Kamloops, apart from those required by his official duties such as the operation of the Tranquille Tuberculosis Society. He devoted considerable energy to his professional life, setting up a training programme in tuberculosis care for nurses, constantly writing reports and memoranda to successive provincial secretaries, and pressuring government authorities to re-organize the delivery of tuberculosis treatment. He was also able to work with governments of both Liberal and Conservative stripes, thereby remaining in charge of Tranquille while others were appointed and fired with each election.

However, these abilities and activities were given scant attention beyond restricted medical and political circles. More noticeable to many people during Lapp's tenure were the social distinctions that emerged. At the top of the social ladder were the medical doctors and their families along with the farm manger, bursar, and a few other senior employees. Maintaining and often cultivating a sense of superiority, this group saw little to criticize in social arrangements that provided them with advantages. Another distinct group was formed by the general employees—kitchen help, laundry workers, farm workers, and orderlies. These distinctions between professional and wage-earning employees were certainly not unique to the sanatorium, but with Lapp's encouragement, they became more pronounced in the 1920s and 1930s at Tranquille. The nurses formed a group unto themselves, though inevitably they had social connections with both the patients and the general employees. Dr. Lapp prohibited social contact between nurses and other employees outside of working hours, specifically forbidding dating. Disciplinary situations arose whenever that prohibition was ignored and subsequently discovered.

Finally, the patients were a separate group entirely. Drawn overwhelmingly from the working population of the province, and for the most part dependent upon social assistance, the patients saw themselves (and were seen by all employees) as distinct from everyone else at Tranquille. Social contact between male and female patients was severely restricted, even to the extent of seating men and women separately in the dining room. However, the common bond of tuberculosis seems to have all but erased social distinctions amongst the patient population, creating in a sense a fellowship of "lungers" united in a struggle for survival. Perhaps inevitably, especially given the nature of the disease, the most common patient complaint was how they were at the mercy of doctors and nurses, maids, and orderlies.

Increasingly, as the years progressed, Dr. Lapp seemed to feel that Tranquille was his own little kingdom. The clearest example of this attitude comes from the year before his resignation. As the sole trustee of the Tranquille School, Lapp without consultation decided to deduct $1.50 from the pay cheques of all sanatorium employees for school purposes. The Department of Education quickly advised him to return the deductions from employees' pay cheques and to go through proper channels.[32] Participation in the volunteer fire department that was formed in 1932 was required of male employees by Dr. Lapp rather than encouraged. Though the necessity of most of his decisions was clear, the methods he employed and the social distance he maintained did little to enable employees to regard him kindly.

In the autumn of 1928, Lapp had an opportunity to visit sanatoria in Europe as part of a group of thirty Canadian medical officials. The tour was sponsored by the Sun Life Insurance Company and the Canadian Tuberculosis Association. Highlights of the three-month tour included visits to the King Edward VII Sanatorium near London, visits to sanatoria in Paris, and the International Congress on Tuberculosis in Rome, which was addressed by Mussolini. Upon returning, Lapp began to press his views on reforming tuberculosis treatment in British Columbia upon his colleagues and the Department of the Provincial Secretary. He urged them to regard Tranquille as a training facility for doctors and nurses, to centralize all tuberculosis work at the sanatorium, and to make Tranquille the administrative centre for tuberculosis treatment for the entire province. By shortening the stay allowed to patients at the same time, he argued the sanatorium would become an educational centre and not simply "a home for incurable cases."[33]

Clearly, Lapp had returned to the philosophical position he had arrived with in 1921, and the one voiced by all previous medical superintendents. They all believed the Tranquille Sanatorium should treat curable patients, not provide extended care for advanced cases of the disease. To continue to do so was to misuse the facility. Delegates to the poorly attended annual meeting of the Canadian Tuberculosis Society, held at Tranquille in 1931, supported him in that view. But if Lapp hoped to change the situation, he was destined to have no more success than his predecessors. To underscore his view, in 1935, Lapp noted the death of a patient who had occupied a bed at the sanatorium for seventeen years.[34]

However, he was partially successful in establishing Tranquille as an educational centre for tuberculosis treatment. The course he proposed for doctors did not win approval, but his proposed training programme for nurses gained the cooperation of hospitals in the lower mainland, Kelowna, Cranbrook, Nelson, and Prince Rupert. Beginning in 1931, they sent their student nurses to Tranquille to take a two-month affiliation course in tuberculosis treatment. Though the additional numbers placed extra pressure on the overcrowded nurses' home, the course the student nurses received from Lapp, Bibby and the medical staff at Tranquille was highly regarded by the affiliated hospitals.

On his other proposals, Lapp made no progress. By 1932, he was insisting that similar centralization in Saskatchewan and Ontario was related to the lower death rates from tuberculosis in those provinces. He argued that failure to act was tantamount to neglect:

> It would be considered brutal, to say the least, for a community to stand by and watch thousands of young people being slowly dragged down to their death without some heroic effort being made to save them. We have this very thing happening in our midst.[35]

Statements such as this echoed the views held many years earlier by Dr. Fagan. And like all of his predecessors, Lapp was referring primarily to the situation of British Columbia's European population. From their ranks, by the mid-1930s, the number of lives claimed by the province's number one killer had fallen to just 52 per 100,000—a figure comparable to, or superior to, the death rate from tuberculosis in any other province in Canada. However, for the groups that remained excluded from treatment at Tranquille and other provincial hospitals, the figures were much more disturbing. The Asian population of the province had a death rate from tuberculosis more than twice that of the European population, while the Native figure was close to twenty times higher. The inclusive death rate from tuberculosis for the province was estimated at approximately 80 per 100,000, significantly higher than the national average of 68.[36]

Finally, in 1934, the new Liberal administration seemed ready to acknowledge that a reorganization of tuberculosis services was needed. Concerned at the death rate from tuberculosis in British Columbia and regretting that a proposed new facility in the lower mainland could not be built due to a lack of money, Provincial Secretary Weir called together medical and provincial officials for a series of conferences. At the Hotel Vancouver in November 1934, Lapp chaired a session on tuberculosis at the Conference on Health and Welfare. Preliminary plans indicated that the entire reorganization was to be coordinated by Dr. Lapp along the lines he had long advocated.[37]

In July 1935, the complete overhaul of tuberculosis services was announced. A Tuberculosis Division under the Provincial Board of Health was created to deal broadly and systematically with what was still the province's number one killer. However, Lapp must have been disappointed. The central administration offices were to be set up in Vancouver, not at Tranquille. Though the 332 beds at the sanatorium represented very nearly half the total available for tuberculosis patients in the province, Vancouver was to become "the hub of the whole anti-tuberculosis drive in British Columbia." The Vancouver Clinic was to be expanded and a forty-bed ward for tuberculosis patients was opened at the Royal Jubilee Hospital in Victoria. Tuberculosis wards specifically for Chinese and Japanese patients were opened, and the Tuberculosis Division agreed to work closely with the Department of Indian Affairs to address the situation with the Native population. No expansion of facilities was announced for Tranquille, though tentative plans for the operating theatre were confirmed. The three treatment centres were to be rather blandly referred to in future as the Vancouver Unit, the Victoria Unit, and the Tranquille Unit.

By the mid-1930s, the superintendent of the Tranquille Unit was becoming less content in the job he had held for a decade and a half. He was honoured by distinctions from both his profession and from society at large. In 1935, he was elected president of the British Columbia Medical Association and was one of the province's recipients of the King George Jubilee medal, an award given to those prominent in public service.[38] From September 1935 to June 1936, he was granted a leave of absence to take his Diploma of Public Health at the University of Toronto. (During his absence, Elizabeth Cooney wrote to the provincial government offering to re-purchase her house and orchard. The government repeated its willingness to see her remain there during her lifetime, but refused to consider her offer to buy.)[39] A cause he had long championed—the reorganization and centralization of tuberculosis care in the province—was achieved, but with neither Tranquille nor himself at the heart.

With another provincial election expected, Lapp decided soon after his return from Toronto that it was time to move on. He advised the provincial secretary he could not face again the turmoil, allegations, and staff disruptions that followed upon the elections of 1928 and 1933. Lapp resigned effective 30 April 1937, ending fifteen years at Tranquille, and soon accepted an appointment as the medical superintendent of the St. Lawrence Sanatorium in Cornwall, Ontario. With his departure, a distinct chapter in the history of the Tranquille Sanatorium ended. A splendid tribute to him by J.R. Pyper had appeared in the last issue of *The Tranquillian* the previous November. The *Kamloops Sentinel*, whose editor J.J. Kerr had recently succeeded Pyper as editor of *The Tranquillian*, quoted extensively from Pyper's article and added its own statement of commendation and regret at seeing such an able man leave the district.[40]

Chapter Notes

1 British Columbia *Sessional Papers* 1922, First Annual Report of the Tranquille Sanatorium, pp. I7-I8.
2 Henry T. Denison, "Health and Happiness for our Disabled Soldiers in the Garden City" (Kamloops, 1920).
3 *The Tranquillian*, November 1920; National Archives of Canada (NAC), MG 28 I 75 volume 12, file 94, Appendix III, pp. 50-54.
4 NAC RG 38, volume 190, file 8635, Denison to Irving, 26 September 1921; Irving to Manion, 28 September 1921; and Denison to DSCR 22 October 1921.
5 NAC, RG 38, volume 190, file 8635.
6 NAC, RG 38, volume 190, file 8635; The Tranquillian, July 1922, pp. 15-6.
7 Eugene Cooney was dismissed from employment shortly afterwards. Other notarized allegations of bad faith are included in the family history. See Eric Norfolk, *Cooney and his Clan*, (Prince George, 1979) pp. 82-97. See also *Kamloops Standard-Sentinel*, 21 November 1922, p. 1. The records of the Anti-Tuberculosis Society contain no reference to a gift of land by Charles Cooney.
8 NAC, RG 38, volume 190, file 8635; *The Tranquillian*, August/November 1925.
9 *Kamloops Sentinel-Standard*, 6 May 1927, p. 1.
10 For those interested in particular organizations and individuals, the pages of *The Tranquillian* from 1919 to 1936 are the most useful source of information, though not all performances and visits are mentioned.
11 British Columbia Archives and Records Service (BCARS), GR 2654, box 1, file 3.
12 BCARS, GR 2866, box 1, file 1, Dr. Irving, "The Early Days of Tranquille"; *The Tranquillian*, August 1921, p. 4. and September 1921, p. 3.
13 Interview with Joan Best, 16 January 1999; BCARS, GR 2654, box 1, file 3.
14 *The Tranquillian*, July 1926, p. 3.
15 British Columbia Lung Association Archives, box 1, Auditor's report, 7 April 1932.
16 British Columbia *Sessional Papers*, First and Second Reports of the Tranquille Sanatorium, 1922 and 1923. The per diem rate was reduced to just 70 cents in 1927 because of the objections of municipal governments, and raised to $1.25 in 1934 over the objections of municipal governments.
17 BCARS, GR 108, box 1, file 3.
18 BCARS, GR 108, box 2, file 3.
19 H.L. Burris, *Medical Saga: The Burris Clinic and Early Pioneers* (Vancouver: 1967); *Victoria Daily Times*, 25 November 1936, p. 13.
20 *Kamloops Sentinel*, 27 October 1925, p. 1; 28 December 1928, p. 1.
21 BCARS, GR 108, box 2, file 6, Lapp to Provincial Secretary, 25 February 1933.
22 British Columbia *Sessional Papers* 1932, Tenth Annual Report on Tranquille; *Kamloops Sentinel*, 23 July 1934, p. 1.
23 BCARS, GR 108, box 1, file 3.
24 BCARS, GR 108, Tranquille Sanatorium, box 2, file 3; box 3, file 7.
25 *Kamloops Sentinel*, 6 May 1927, p. 2.

26 *The Tranquillian*, August 1931, p. 14.
27 Vancouver Sun, 16 August 1935, p. 10. When the provincial government developed its "representative Indian village" across from the Crystal gardens in 1940, the stone basin was removed to Victoria. (BCARS, GR 108, Deputy Provincial Secretary to H.S. Stalker, 3 September 1940.)
28 BCARS, GR 497, box 8, file 4, Lapp to Walker, 10 June 1932.
29 BCARS, GR 108, box 2, file 3; British Columbia *Sessional Papers* 1933, Eleventh Annual Report of the Tranquille Sanatorium, p. O6; BCARS, GR 2654, British Columbia, Department of the Provincial Secretary, box 1, file 6.
30 *Kamloops Sentinel*, 27 February 1934, p. 1.
31 *Kamloops Sentinel*, 24 July 1934, p. 1. Lost in the midst of all this political wrangling was the news that Dr. Procter, the former medical health officer at the Royal Inland Hospital who had sought to establish the sanatorium in Kamloops in 1901, had been murdered in Vancouver by a disgruntled CPR employee.
32 The Tranquille School was unlike any other in the province. The Thompson Valley School District, which governed it, levied no taxes and was therefore unaudited. After the early 1920s, it was essentially run by a single trustee, namely the superintendent of the Tranquille Sanatorium. Like other rural schools with low enrolment, rules were sometimes bent. One September, for example, Dr. Lapp permitted three under-age children to register in order to prevent the school from having to close. (Bette Wood Interview, 3 November 1998) With few students from elsewhere, most of the clientele of the school were the children of sanatorium employees. A new schoolhouse was built in 1923, but the small school suffered from the same inability to retain staff, as did the rest of the sanatorium; teachers typically had little previous experience and usually stayed two years at most. However, the school achieved almost annual distinction after the appointment in 1929 of Beverley Fyfe, who remained for several years. His abilities resulted in regular awards at the Yale-Cariboo Music Festival for the twelve to fifteen students under his instruction.
33 British Columbia Lung Association Archives, box 1, David Alexander Stewart, "Travel Notes: European Tour of Canadian Doctors Associated with Tuberculosis Sanatoria and Clinics, September-October 1928"; British Columbia *Sessional Papers* 1932, Ninth Report on the Tranquille Sanatorium 1929-30, p. V5.
34 NAC, MG 28, I75, volume 4, file 11, Lapp to G.J. Wherrett, 2 March 1935.
35 British Columbia *Sessional Papers* 1933. Eleventh Report on the Tranquille Sanatorium 1931-2, p. O5.
36 NAC, MG 28 I75, volume 4, file 11, Confidential Memorandum on Tuberculosis Policy, Department of the Provincial Secretary, 19 December 1934.
37 NAC, MG 28 I 75, volume 4, file 11, Confidential Memorandum on Tuberculosis Policy, Department of the Provincial Secretary, 19 December 1934.
38 Other recipients associated with Tranquille were Blanche Bibby, J.R. Pyper, and the chaplain Reverend E.D. McLaren.
39 BCARS, GR 108, box 4, file 2.
40 *Kamloops Sentinel*, 16 April 1937, pp. 1-2; *The Tranquillian*, November 1936, p. 15.

An Institution in its Prime: 1937-1952

The resignation of Dr. Lapp led to the first smooth transition in management in the history of the sanatorium. Unlike the situations when Irving and Vrooman resigned, the Tranquille institution was not in a state of turmoil and uncertainty, and there was no series of short-lived or temporary appointments before a satisfactory successor was found. Mindful of Lapp's persistent recommendations, the provincial government sought a man who, above all else, was a capable administrator. With little hesitation, a decision was made. Herbert Stewart Stalker was a graduate of the University of Manitoba. He came to British Columbia in 1928 and was the assistant superintendent at Vancouver General Hospital at the time of his appointment. He would remain as superintendent at Tranquille for precisely as long as had Dr. Lapp—fifteen years. Doctor Stalker began his duties at Tranquille on 17 May 1937, joining the newly appointed matron, Gladys Currie.

The New Regime

Essentially, the conditions under which the sanatorium operated did not change with the arrival of the new supervisors. Filled to capacity, the institution had seen little development during the decade since 1928, and further construction was not contemplated at the time of Stalker's appointment. Nevertheless, soon after Stalker's arrival, two improvements approved during the latter stages of Lapp's superintendence were accomplished. Contaminating bacteria were twice detected in the water supply during the summer of 1936, and after August 1937, the drinking water of the sanatorium was chlorinated. After years of delay, a complete operating theatre was finally opened on the third floor of the Greaves Building by Lieutenant Governor Eric Hamber in September 1938. As the institution still lacked surgical staff, Dr. J.S. Burris visited weekly, but it was no longer necessary to require Tranquille patients to travel to Kamloops for major operations.

Though the stability of the institution was unaffected by the change of superintendents, Stalker did not simply adopt the style and methods of his predecessor. In significant respects, he was specifically instructed by the office of the provincial secretary not to do so. For example, he was asked to improve the relations between the institution and the community of Kamloops. Soon after his arrival, Stalker quickly became familiar with the delicate nature of the relationship between Kamloops and the institution when some city merchants complained to the provincial secretary that the Canteen was undermining their ability to do business. Whereas Lapp avoided contact with Kamloops, Stalker cultivated it. He attended church in the city, and joined the Rotary Club and several other organizations. Just two months after his arrival, when the opportunity presented itself to take part in Kamloops' 125th anniversary celebrations, Stalker did not hesitate to involve the institution. The farm truck was decorated to look like a ship and was named the *SS Good Health*. Four nurses in uniform and a number of Tranquille school children dressed as sailors waved to onlookers as the vehicle took its place in the parade.

Stalker was also advised by the provincial secretary to improve relations with employees and to diminish the social stratification that had been encouraged by Dr. Lapp. This could not be accomplished quickly, but Stalker made a point of entertaining employees in his home during the first few years of his appointment in order to break down what he described as the "social barriers previously imposed." Staff and patients alike welcomed their Sunday afternoon encounters with Stalker and his wife, Irma, as the pair strolled about the hospital grounds and the farm.[1] The process was assisted by the arrival of Dr. Evelyn Gee. A patient at Tranquille in 1939, Gee became the first woman doctor appointed to the institution in 1941. She performed the first pneumolysis operation at Tranquille in 1942. Her outgoing personality and the art classes she offered over the years to staff also contributed to the new atmosphere of collegiality.

The problem of staff retention was partially addressed by the introduction of the standard 48-hour work week for most employees of the provincial government, a proposal that, happily for Dr. Stalker, coincided with his arrival. By early 1938, Stalker was pleased to report that all employees with the exception of the nursing staff were working 48 hours per week. Provincial budget priorities of the 1930s did not include funds to hire the additional nurses that would have been required. A motion presented by the CCF to bring nurses within the 48-hour limit by limiting their workdays to eight-hours was defeated in the provincial legislature in late 1938. The situation of non-medical support staff stabilized to some extent because of the reduction in the work week, but the difficulty in maintaining sufficient numbers of nurses remained. Long hours in conditions of relative isolation continued to make Tranquille unattractive to most young single nurses, while the complete absence of appropriate accommodation meant married nurses had little opportunity to become employees at the sanatorium. The disease itself also discouraged many nurses from entering the field of tuberculosis work. Though Tranquille pointed with pride to its own record, there were always several nurses from other hospitals at Tranquille as patients.

Other regulations governing employees also received Stalker's attention. The prohibition on nurses dating orderlies, for example, was lifted soon after Stalker's arrival, and employees who volunteered for the fire department were given a small token payment for their services beginning in 1938. Other changes were examined as necessary responses to the ongoing employment problems. All full-time employees were required to live at Tranquille, but the existing accommodation was grossly inadequate. Within weeks of assuming his responsibilities, Stalker wrote to the Director of the Tuberculosis Control Branch that even the doctors' apartments were "little short of appalling." He described the charge of $42.50 per month for rent of the small apartments, with their paper-thin walls and noisy plumbing, as a definite factor in the "dissatisfaction felt by the medical staff." He noted that a few non-medical employees were still living in the tarpaper shacks purchased by the British Columbia Anti-Tuberculosis Society after the railway construction of 1912. Stalker urged that serious attention be paid to wage rates and, realizing that the construction of additional accommodation was unlikely during depressed economic times, suggested that employees be permitted to live in Kamloops.

Both suggestions received approval after the outbreak of the war added to the difficulties of retaining competent staff. With a guarantee of returning to their jobs after the war, many young male employees joined the armed forces, and staff turnover increased sharply. Women took over many tasks previously denied them, but the extra female staff added new accommodation pressures. The Maids' Home was so overcrowded by 1940 that one of the cure cottages in front of the Greaves Building had to be used for accommodation. By early 1942, certain married employees were permitted to live in Kamloops and Stalker noted that the sixteen married men who did so were among the institution's "most reliable" staff. Within a few months, policy was changed to permit nurses to live away from Tranquille, and married nurses resident in Kamloops thereby became eligible for employment at Tranquille. Most of the employees who lived in Kamloops took advantage of the bus service that was offered by BC Coach Lines, while a very few drove private automobiles. The daily commute that would become such a regular feature for so many residents of Kamloops had begun.

In other respects, too, the war furthered the integration of Tranquille with the wider world. The renewed need to finance a war saw the return of Victory Bonds. Contributions from Tranquille to all eight Victory Loan campaigns were high, a fact that undoubtedly pleased the Kamloops-area chair of the National War Finance Committee in charge of the campaigns—former superintendent Robert Irving. Many patients contributed more than money. The Kamloops Red Cross asked if patients would be willing to join its campaign to knit for the forces overseas. The opportunity was provided by the occupational therapy classes, available at the institution again after 1939 under the guidance of Madge Farmer. Twenty-seven women patients agreed to help, providing the Red Cross in the first six months of the war with dozens of gloves, billfolds, tobacco pouches, and even one large bible cover.[2]

If the integration of Tranquille with the outside world seemed to have been achieved, in some respects the administration at the sanatorium may have preferred the earlier isolation. In May 1940, Stalker advised W.H. Hatfield of "Soviet activities at the Tranquille Unit." As many as twenty-two employees were named by Stalker, and copies of the periodical *Soviet Russia Today* were said to be widely circulated. Kamloops MLA R.H. Carson called for an investigation of subversive activities at the sanatorium and an undercover RCMP investigation was undertaken. The RCMP was also called upon when cocaine, heroin, and liquid opium were stolen from the pharmacy at the sanatorium in June 1943. Kamloops' four known drug users were the prime suspects.[3]

By late 1942, wage increases for dietary and cleaning staff were approved in a further attempt to reduce the high staff turnover and to counter the growing interest in the formation of an employees' union. The administration expressed concern at the first attempts by Tranquille employees to form a branch of the Provincial Employees' Association in July 1943. Nurses also felt the need to organize and by 1944, the Tranquille-Kamloops branch of the British Columbia Registered Nurses Association had been established.[4] Before the formation of their association, nurses were finally granted the 48-hour work week. In 1942, their wages were increased to nearly $90 per month plus room, board, and laundry services valued at $27.50 per month. This made Tranquille nurses the highest paid in the province.

However, the isolation of the institution and the general shortage throughout the province kept the number of graduate nurses at Tranquille at a critically low level. The elimination of the affiliation course for student nurses after 1943 revealed the extent to which the institution had come to depend on their labour. In April 1939, Vancouver General Hospital began to offer its own course and the number of student nurses taking the course at Tranquille fell significantly. The affiliation course was offered by the Tuberculosis Division in Vancouver after 1944 and the course at Tranquille was cancelled. Since 1931, when the training course was first offered, patients at the institution had been attended by thirty graduate nurses, who could count on the assistance of as many as a dozen student nurses. Requiring a minimum of forty-four nurses after the opening of the operating theatre in 1938, the institution felt the loss of the student nurses profoundly. The number of nurses employed at the institution declined steadily during 1942, reaching just thirty-three by the end of the year. A rumour that all nurses in the province were to be frozen in their positions at the end of April resulted in seven resignations. The closure of wards was seriously contemplated during 1942 and 1943 because of the nursing shortage.

The condition of the nurses' home had long been a source of concern. By late 1940, the building was accommodating sixty-one nurses, student nurses and nurses' aides, but only by doubling up in several rooms and only after the graduate nurses' sitting room had been converted into a dormitory for four. Stalker advised the Director of the Tuberculosis Control Branch: "A practice of having nurses who are working with tuberculosis patients sharing small bedrooms is bad and I would very much like to have this changed." He listed the inadequacies as follows: inadequate toilet facilities, no dining room, no laundry facilities, no separate accommodation for night nurses, small and unsatisfactory kitchens and no place to study for affiliate nurses-in-training.[5] He recommended the construction of a second nurses' home to accommodate thirty nurses at a cost of $45,000. Without it, he argued, the sanatorium would continue to face difficulty in attracting and retaining capable nursing staff. Despite Stalker's concern, the sanatorium would see no change in nurses' accommodation for the remainder of the decade. The cancellation of the nurses' affiliation course at Tranquille in 1943 and, ironically, the continuing shortage of graduate nurses willing to work there combined to relieve the pressure on space in the existing nurses' home. By the end of 1944, in fact, there was no pressure on accommodation in the nurses' home as numbers fell to fewer than thirty.

Construction at Tranquille increased during the war years. Some of the balconies in the Main and the Infirmary buildings were enclosed in 1940, enabling the capacity of the institution to increase to nearly 350 beds. The demolition of the Cooney ranch house was ordered in 1941, soon after the death of Elizabeth Cooney at the age of ninety-six. The task was soon accomplished by sanatorium ranch hands, and the land was added to the alfalfa acreage.[6] The most significant construction was that of the long-awaited multi-purpose auditorium. The IODE demonstrated its continuing support of the institution by assisting with construction costs, as did the Canteen Fund, the Vancouver Kinsmen Club, and the British Columbia Tuberculosis Society (successor to the Tranquille Tuberculosis Society). Together they paid for approximately forty percent of the cost of the building. Opened in March 1941 by Rocky Mountain Ranger Major A.P. Williams, the Tranquille Hall immediately became the social centre for the entire community of both staff and patients. The weekly movies for staff and patients were shown there instead of in the Main

Building. The auditorium also served as a dance hall and indoor sports facility, while a kitchen, small rooms for bridge parties, showers, and a staff library were also part of the complex. The opening procedures were broadcast to the entire institution over the sanatorium's radio system, and Tranquille fire chief George "Chuck" Sealy created a large tropical scene as a stage backdrop.

Whether due to Stalker's involvement in the community of Kamloops, whether the decision to allow Tranquille workers to live in Kamloops was having an effect, or whether the city was simply maturing, the local region's attitude to Tranquille continued to improve. Symbolic of the new attitude was a speech Dr. Irving made to the local Rotary Club in March 1943. At the head table with him was eighty-seven-year-old W.W. Shaw, the first ranch superintendent employed by the Anti-Tuberculosis Society in 1907. Irving did not refer to his bitterness of years ago or to the controversies of the more recent past. Instead he detailed the struggles of the first few years and paid tribute to the work of the modern institution on the lake that had become an accepted part of the Kamloops region. Due to the advent of the Coalition Liberal-Conservative government in British Columbia after 1941, the traditional local political rivalries and the petty criticisms so common before the war also diminished considerably. Political criticism was supplied by the CCF, which frequently criticized working conditions and class distinctions at the institution.

In 1944, the government acknowledged that provincial facilities were inadequate for the treatment of the growing number of tuberculosis victims and announced plans to construct a new 250-bed tuberculosis hospital. The Kamloops Board of Trade lost little time in adopting the position that the new hospital should be located adjacent to the existing Tranquille facilities. It sent a delegation, which included businessman Syd Smith and Dr. Irving, to Victoria to meet with the provincial cabinet. Not for the first time, all the benefits of the dry Interior climate were drawn to the attention of decision-makers.[7] Clearly, four decades of proximity to the institution at Tranquille had eradicated fears of contamination and made obvious the economic advantages to the community of Kamloops. The payroll by the end of World War II exceeded $300,000. The cabinet agreed to consider the views of the delegation, but announced soon afterwards that the new facility would be built in the lower mainland.

Tranquille Farm: Problems and Progress

The political upheaval anticipated by Lapp did not occur after the provincial election of 1937 because the governing party did not change. Nevertheless, the Liberal administration decided again to enquire into the operations of the sanatorium. An auditor arrived in late 1938 (causing the usual flurry of interest and speculation in Kamloops), with special instructions to scrutinize the farm operation. Farm Manager Davis, like his predecessor, was giving much of his time and attention to the beef herd, and a year after his appointment, he was also able to pursue his related academic interests. Adjacent to Tranquille, an experimental farm had been opened by the federal Department of Agriculture in 1935, located there specifically because the laboratory at the sanatorium could provide the facilities required for research. With Lapp's encouragement, the provincial government had agreed to the arrangement, and the sanatorium farm cooperated with the experimental farm in efforts to improve stock and methods of weed control. For experimental purposes, up to forty of the sanatorium's Hereford cattle were kept at Pass Lake. However, with Lapp's departure, the government became cool to the idea and soon sought to end its association with the experimental farm. The slow decline in the swine and dairy herds throughout the decade was seen as a consequence of the concentration on beef, and the government demanded a hard-nosed assessment of the whole farm operation.

Pete Moore, in charge of the Colony Farm at Essondale, was sent to Tranquille in February 1940 to provide that assessment. Ironically, this was not Moore's first investigation of the farm operation at Tranquille. In 1919, he had been asked to visit Tranquille for precisely the same reasons. He was not at all impressed by the condition of the dairy herd under Strachan in 1919, and he was not impressed by the dairy herd under the stewardship of Davis in 1940. He attributed the decline in the swine and dairy herds directly to the farm manager's inclination to focus upon what he knew best: beef. Moore acknowledged that Davis had improved the cattle operation immensely. In fact, the sanatorium now had a herd that was greater than its needs demanded. However, he also noted that the once great dairy herd of Holsteins and Friesians was reduced to just forty-six animals, eighteen of which were dry. The swine, he commented, would become “an absolute menace to the Sanatorium” when the heat of summer returned. He suggested the piggery be located further from the institution. He urged the deputy provincial secretary to end the experimental arrangements permanently, especially considering that, by the time of his visit, the federal authorities had halted the project temporarily due to war priorities. He further suggested that the beef requirements of the institution could be more economically met by the open market than by maintaining its own beef herd. Sale of the entire beef herd and a renewed concentration on dairy and swine were recommended. Davis was displeased, and was even more displeased in April when Moore was appointed senior supervisor of the government farms at both Essondale and Tranquille.[8]

The government acted quickly on nearly all Moore’s recommendations. The dairy herd was bolstered by ten cows sent up from Essondale’s Colony Farm. Much to the annoyance of the federal government, the arrangement with the experimental station was unilaterally cancelled in late April. The announcement was made in June that almost the entire herd of Hereford cattle was to be auctioned in Kamloops as soon as arrangements could be made. Sufficient cattle to satisfy the institution’s needs until 1942 were to be retained, after which time the sanatorium would purchase its beef on the open market. Davis voiced his objections, but was reluctant to alter his methods and priorities at the farm. His resignation was accepted by the provincial government in August 1940.

The federal government and Davis were not the only ones displeased. The Kamloops Board of Trade protested the sale in a letter to Provincial Secretary Weir in June. It was joined by protests from the Nicola Stock Breeders Association, the Douglas Lake Cattle Company, and the British Columbia Beef Cattle Growers Association. All were concerned that such a large auction of high-grade beef could affect cattle prices, giving an advantage to a large operator able to purchase the cattle as a single lot. Though fifty head were sold separately to Pat Burns and Company, the government met the objections by agreeing to sell the remainder in smaller lots. Plans went forward with notices appearing in newspapers throughout the province, and on 31 October 1940, the Kamloops stockyards auctioned nearly 700 Hereford cattle from the sanatorium ranch. The prices fetched were high, but many local cattlemen took the opportunity to strengthen their herds. After expenses were deducted, more than $32,000 had been raised at auction. When added to the revenue from the Burns purchase, more than $35,000 found its way into the province's general revenues.[9]

The money was set aside for farm improvements at Tranquille. Though six teams of horses continued to leave the barn every morning ready for work, their days were numbered. The first tractor and bulldozer were soon added to the equipment of the farm. With the renewed focus on the dairy herd, the construction of a pasteurization plant was approved in 1941. The milk requirements of the sanatorium stood at 80,000 gallons annually by the early war years, and while constant testing had revealed only occasional problems, the new plant ensured that safety and quality would be maintained. A new modern dairy was also constructed during the summer of 1942. Its completion coincided with the withdrawal of the Tranquille farm from large-scale beef operation. The leases on 275 acres of grazing lands were not renewed. However, these lands were set aside as the Tranquille Sanatorium Reserve so residents would be protected from any use of the land incompatible with the sanatorium's purposes. Though a small beef herd would remain, the conversion to a focus on the dairy herd was complete. Overseeing the conversion to dairy production was a new farm manager. Robert Sutton, from the provincial Department of Agriculture, was appointed on Moore's recommendation in November 1940. However, he was unable to continue after the spring of 1942 due to ill health, and an acting farm manager was appointed in his place.

Just a year later, a cannery was opened at the farm next to the dairy barn. Well equipped with a boiler, juice extractor, juice press, a syrup vat, capper, and a retort oven, the cannery had a capacity of three to five hundred U.S. gallon cans daily. Soon it was providing canned tomatoes, Swiss chard and other vegetables, cherries and apple juice. While it supplied the sanatorium with most of its needs, it also required a seasonal workforce. The workers were drawn from the same labour pool in Kamloops as the nurses' aides, maids, and kitchen help. In its first few years of operation, some staff were transferred temporarily to the cannery, causing an additional strain on the ability of the sanatorium to operate at full capacity in the late summer and the early fall.

On 10 December 1942, a fire destroyed the building that housed the fire hall, canteen, and ambulance station. The blaze threatened to spread to other buildings, and the volunteer crew at Tranquille required the assistance of the Kamloops fire department to bring the fire under control. Within a year, a new canteen had been constructed, and a new fire hall was opened and equipped with an American-LaFrance fire truck to replace the one lost in the fire.[10]

Several months later, in a daring night-time raid, Dr. Stalker and a government official found a senior farm employee selling farm meat to the owner of a grocery in Kamloops. The culprits were each subsequently sentenced to one year's imprisonment in March 1944. However, the trial provided the kind of publicity no institution or government could welcome. The episode eventually led to the dismissal of the acting farm manager, and Pete Moore again temporarily took over supervisory responsibilities for the farm at Tranquille. Concerned that theft could be a continuing problem, the government set up a separate business office for the farm for the first time early in 1944. Provincial officials visited frequently over the next several months before they were satisfied that the office was indeed being run competently by Gerry Rositch, a young graduate of St. Ann's Academy in Kamloops.[11]

After another short-lived appointment as farm manager proved unsatisfactory, the government followed Pete Moore's advice and placed the herdsman from Colony Farm in charge at Tranquille early in 1947. Like all his predecessors, David Caldow found the operation he had inherited unsatisfactory in certain respects. Caldow complained that not only were the farm workers too numerous, they also gathered the hay improperly and were reluctant to learn new methods. He found the existing irrigation methods inefficient and succeeded in having a new sprinkler system installed. He was also pleased that he was able to convince Kamloops MLA Syd Smith that a new piggery was essential in order to save the institution from the problems of soil contamination. The new piggery was built in 1951 north of the railway, and the old piggery was converted into the abattoir. Caldow's wife Peggy often supervised the seasonal and part-time garden and cannery workers, several of whom were Japanese women from North Kamloops. Their employment by Caldow represented the end of the Asian exclusion from employment at Tranquille that had been in effect since 1919. Though his relations with the Tranquille branch of the British Columbia Government Employees' Association were not always harmonious, Caldow brought a stability to the ranch operation that had been missing since the resignation of Davis in 1940.

The Post-war Years

The end of the war brought little immediate change to the Tranquille patient population. They continued to be served by what one newspaper described approvingly as a "white-coated gentle-footed staff."[12] Undoubtedly, they continued to long for release from the institution and their disease. The influx of tubercular soldiers did occur, but it was not as great as expected and it did not overwhelm the hospital facilities either of the country or of Tranquille as it had in 1919. This was largely because the armed forces systematically x-rayed potential recruits and existing troops, and because battle conditions during the Second World War were less conducive to the spread of tuberculosis than they had been during the First World War. By 1946, there were eighty-five veterans in residence at Tranquille, occupying one-fourth of the beds. The facility was certainly filled to capacity, but this had been the case for many years. The Shaughnessy military hospital in Vancouver was able to accommodate the majority of soldier cases.

Staffing difficulties continued, complicated by returning veterans. Many claimed the right to return to the jobs held at the time of their enlistment, and a certain amount of "bumping" occurred. Due to a combination of the restlessness and optimism of the immediate post-war years, staff turnover remained high, but with the exception of the nurses and kitchen workers, staff shortages apparently were not a problem. Though the attendant difficulties of administration were considerable, Dr. Stalker was relieved of at least one responsibility in the spring of 1946, as the Tranquille School became part of the newly organized Kamloops School District. Though the small school would continue to operate for another twelve years, the medical superintendent of the Tranquille Sanatorium would no longer be required to act as school trustee.

The end of the war did not bring relief to the problem of the shortage of nurses. In fact, staff shortages comparable to those experienced at the end of the First World War were repeated. With 350 patients in residence in June 1946, the number of nurses fell to just twenty-three—barely a third of the full complement of sixty-six the institution required. Just one nurse per floor was available on each shift, and there was no weekend relief. Ward aides and maids were required to take on some of the tasks normally performed by nurses. So serious was the shortage of nurses that a public appeal was issued. Nurses available for employment at Tranquille were asked immediately to telephone Esther Paulson, the superintendent of nurses for the Tuberculosis Division.[13]

Finally convinced that inadequate accommodation was part of the problem, the government several times called for tenders for a project that was to include a new nurses' home, four doctors' residences and a library. However, it could not find a contractor willing to submit a satisfactorily firm bid within government spending limits. The government was applying a new policy in all its construction projects of accepting only bids "with no qualifying clauses whatsoever." Many construction projects were postponed as a result, and the Tranquille project was one of those affected.

Two years later, as the contract remained unlet, the situation of the nurses remained, in the opinion of Dr. Stalker, "desperate." A contractor was finally found, but news that he would not proceed with the proposed new nurses' home after all due to a financial dispute with the government led to resignation of several nurses in April. With fewer than thirty nurses remaining on staff, Stalker commented that the situation was worse than that during the latter war years and again feared that wards would have to be closed. All chest surgery was halted for a time in 1947 and was resumed in 1948 only after auxiliary staff had been further trained to perform more of the tasks usually assigned to nurses. The shortage of nurses eased considerably by January 1948 with forty-one nurses on staff at the sanatorium, but several were commuting from Kamloops because there was no living accommodation for married nurses at the sanatorium.[14]

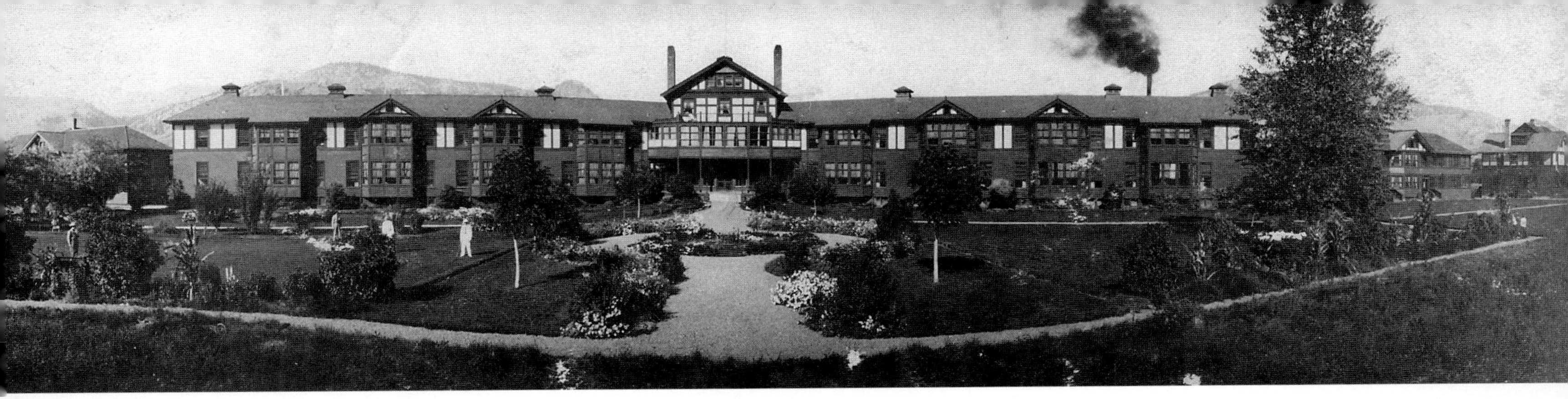

Main Building, 1918
(Courtesy KMA 8611)

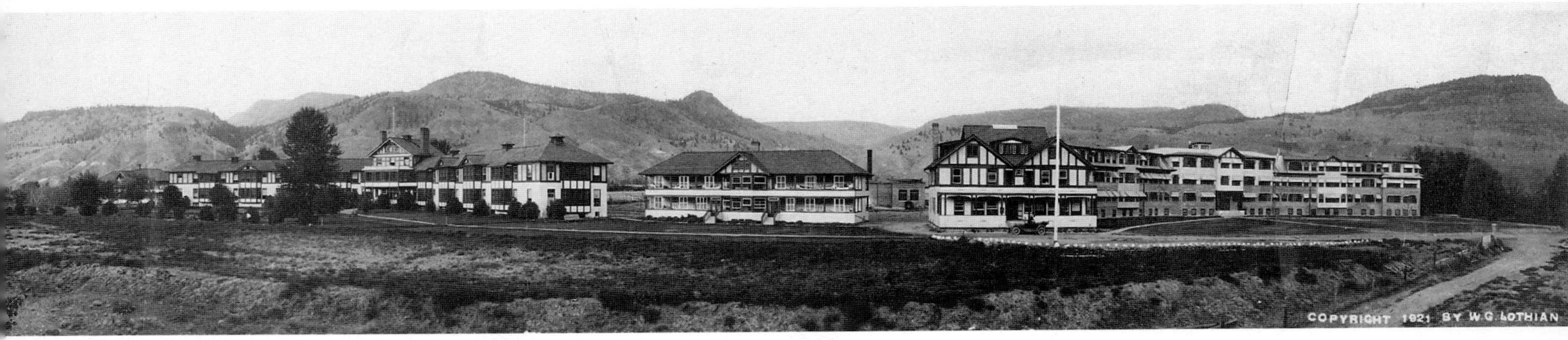

Tranquille Sanatorium, 1921
(Courtesy KMA 8753)

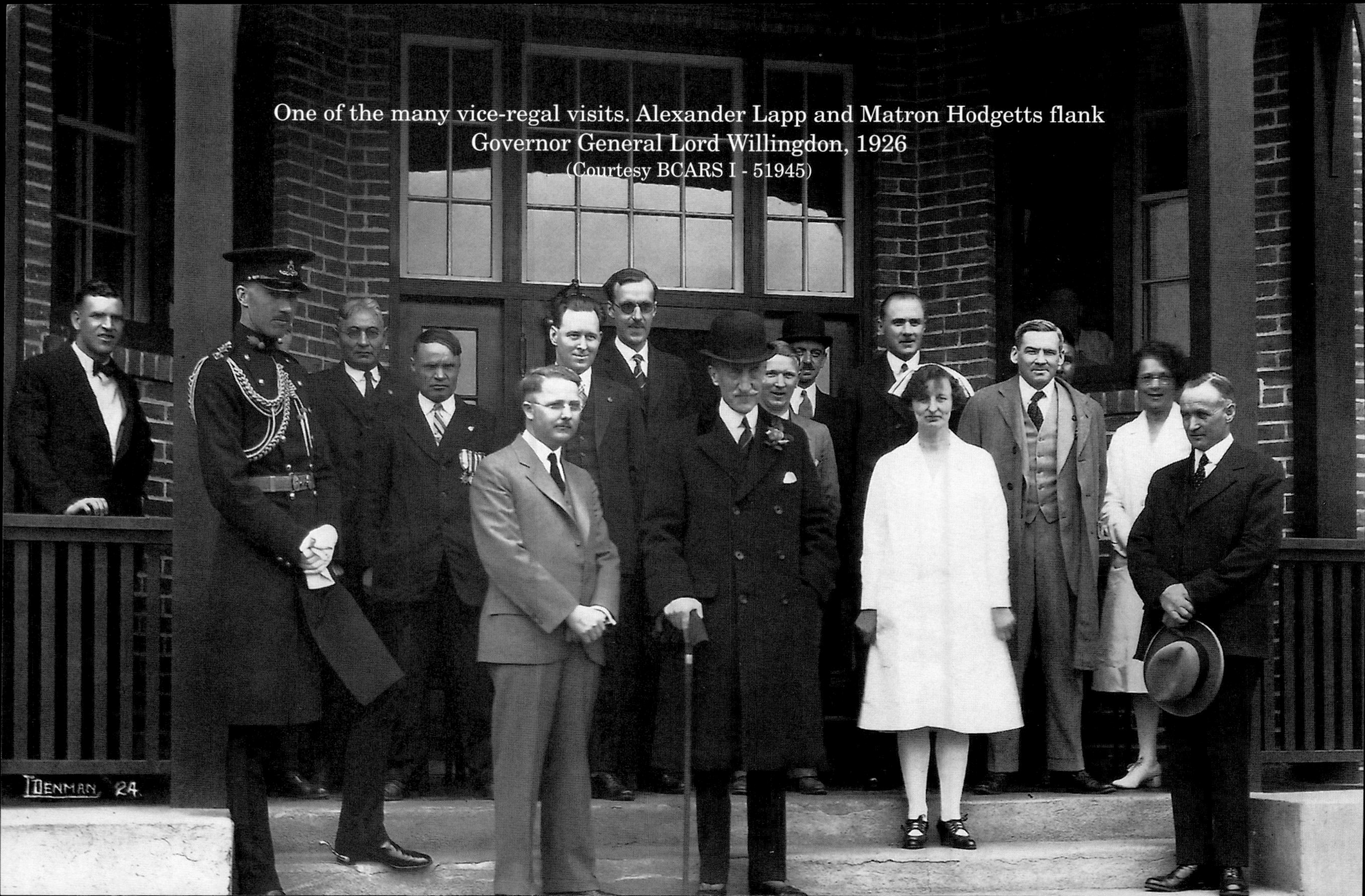

One of the many vice-regal visits. Alexander Lapp and Matron Hodgetts flank Governor General Lord Willingdon, 1926
(Courtesy BCARS I - 51945)

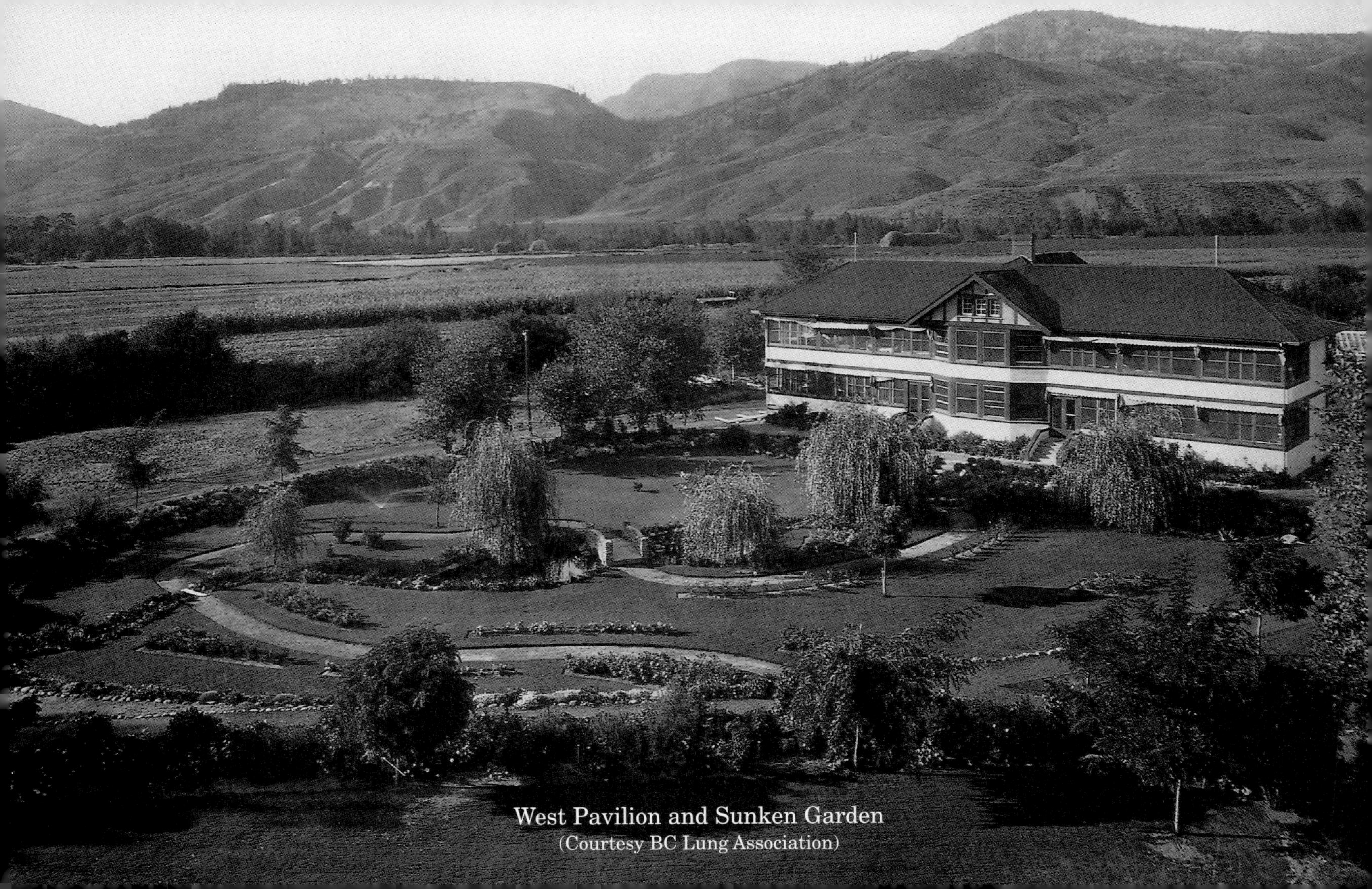

West Pavilion and Sunken Garden
(Courtesy BC Lung Association)

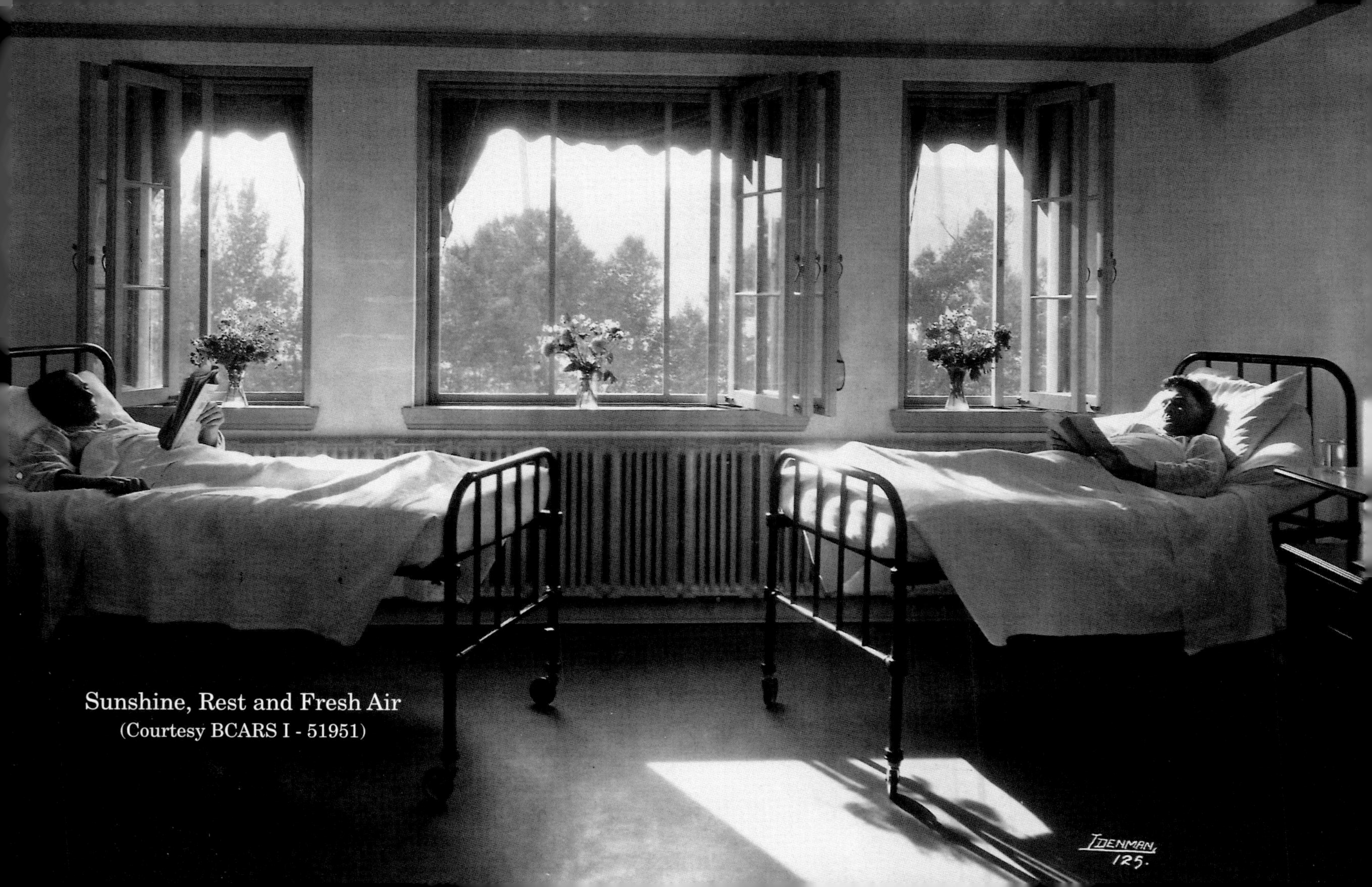

Sunshine, Rest and Fresh Air
(Courtesy BCARS I - 51951)

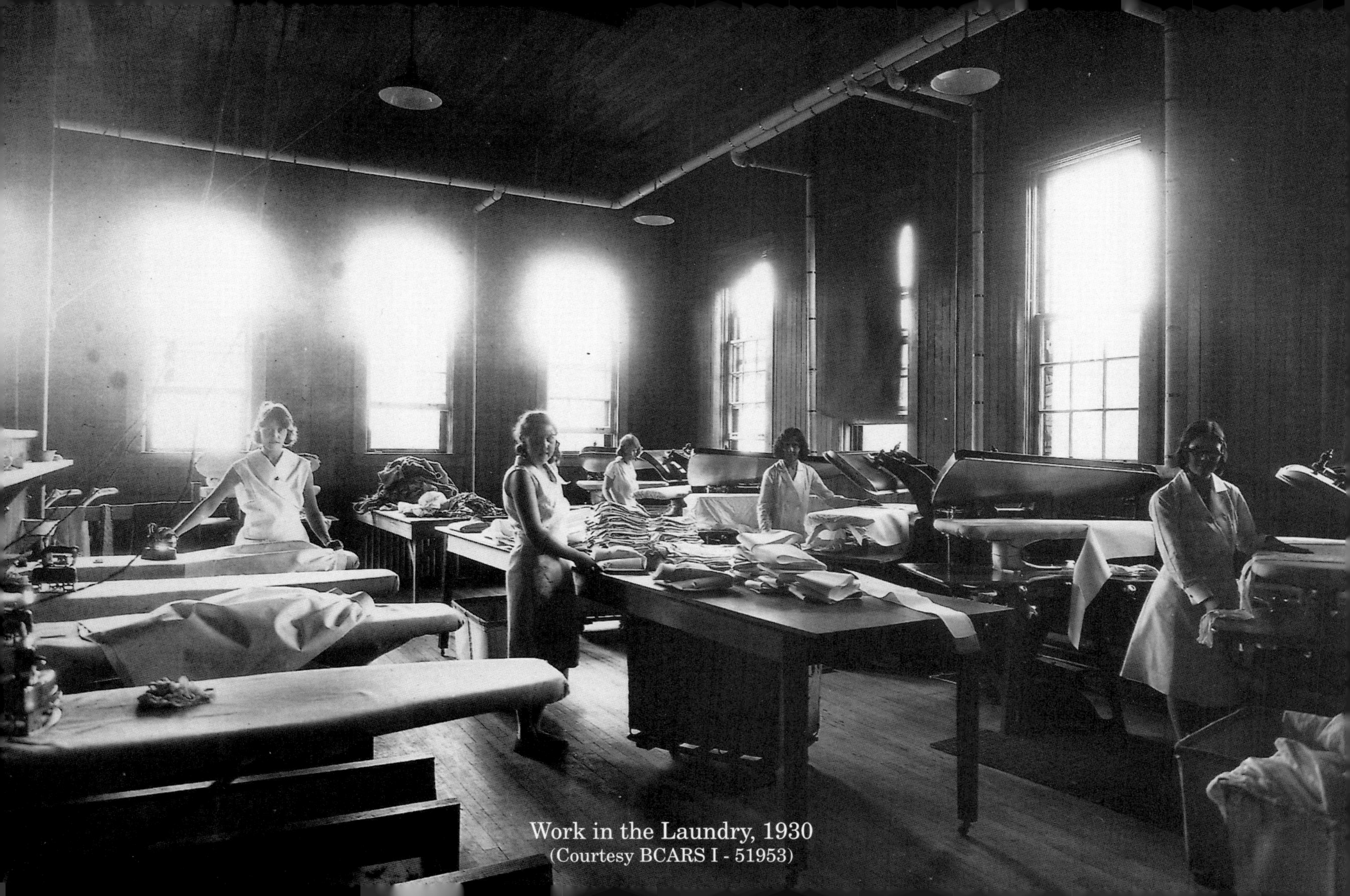

Work in the Laundry, 1930
(Courtesy BCARS I - 51953)

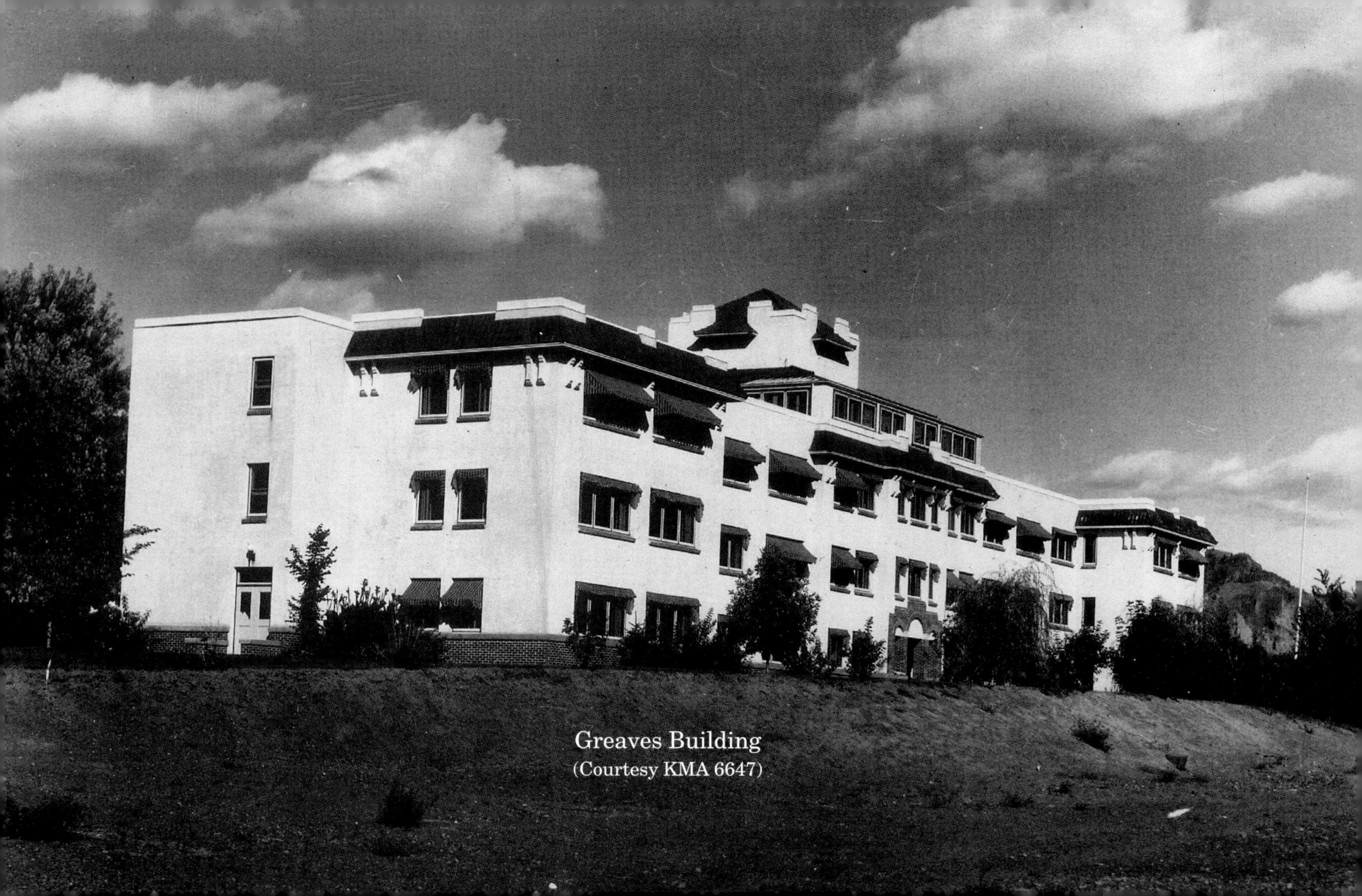

Greaves Building
(Courtesy KMA 6647)

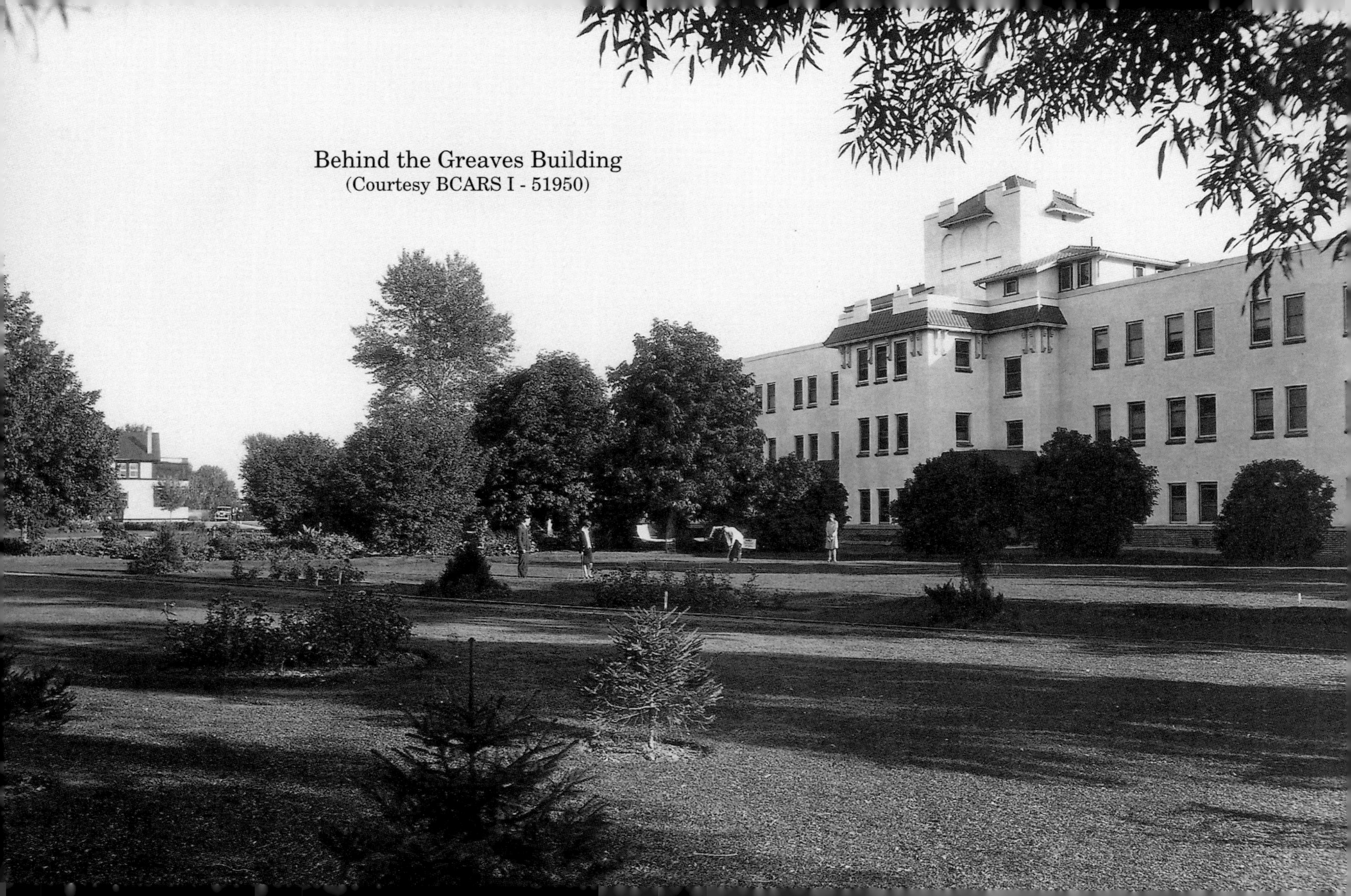

Behind the Greaves Building
(Courtesy BCARS I - 51950)

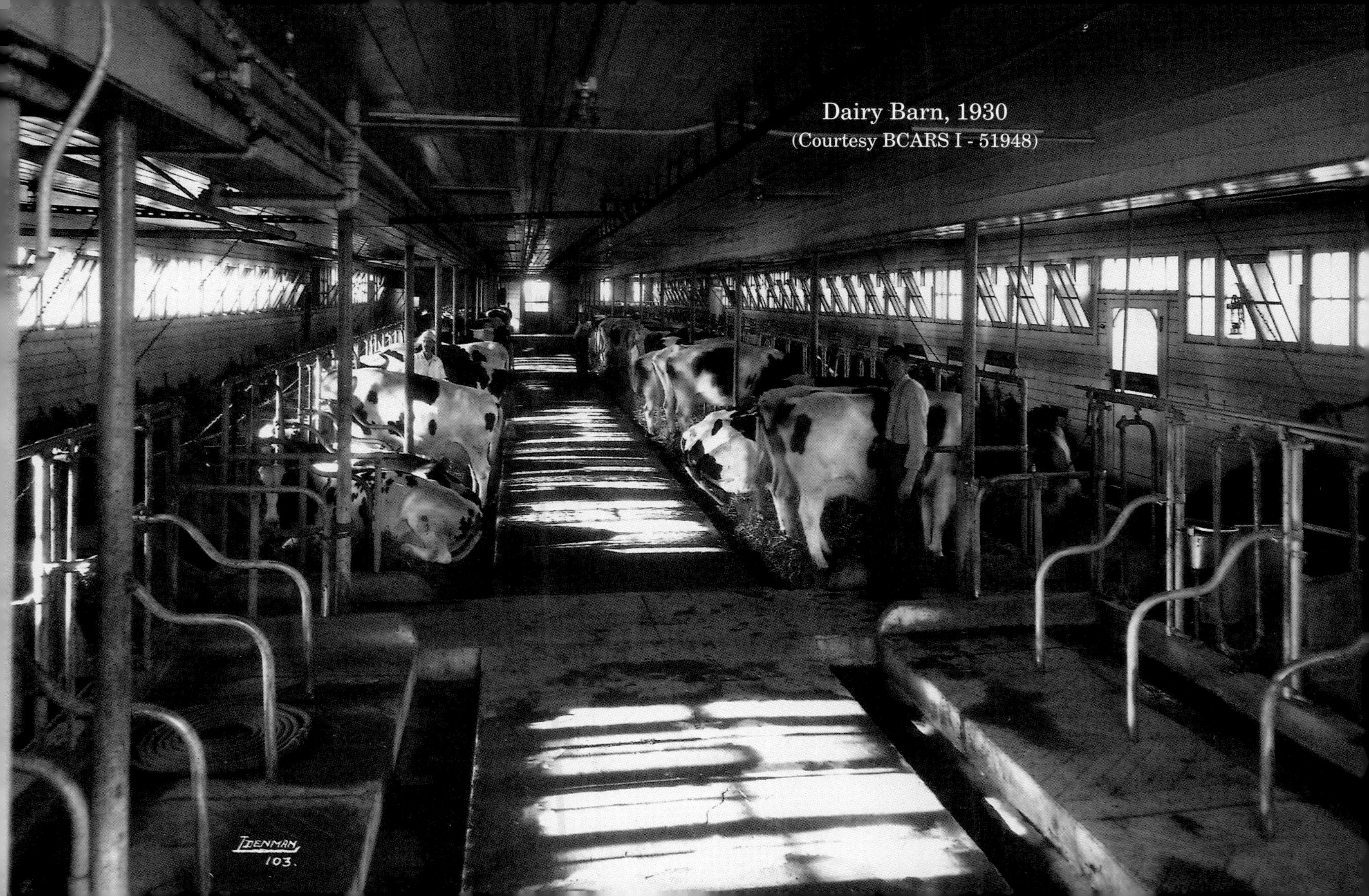

Dairy Barn, 1930
(Courtesy BCARS I - 51948)

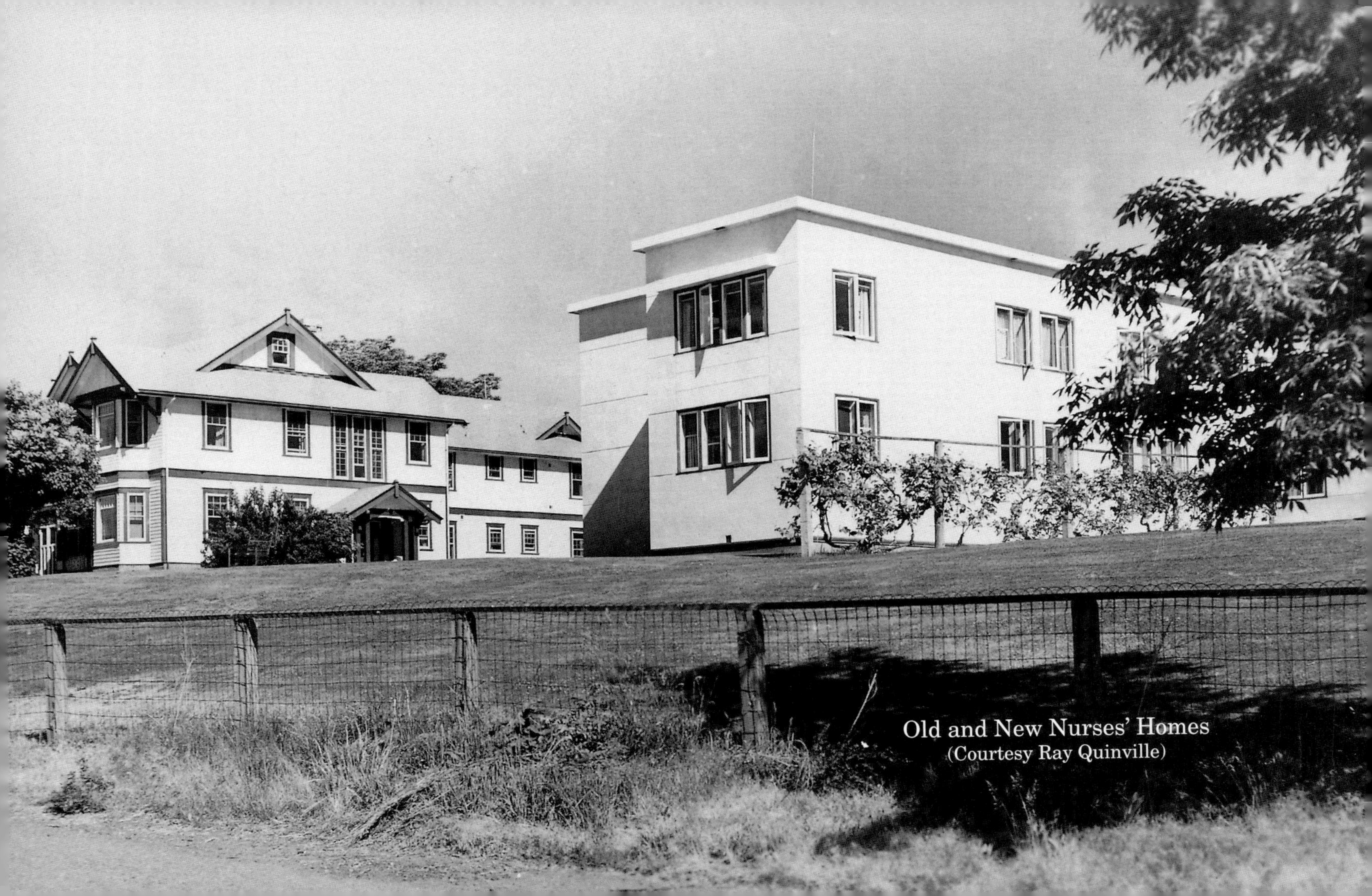

Old and New Nurses' Homes
(Courtesy Ray Quinville)

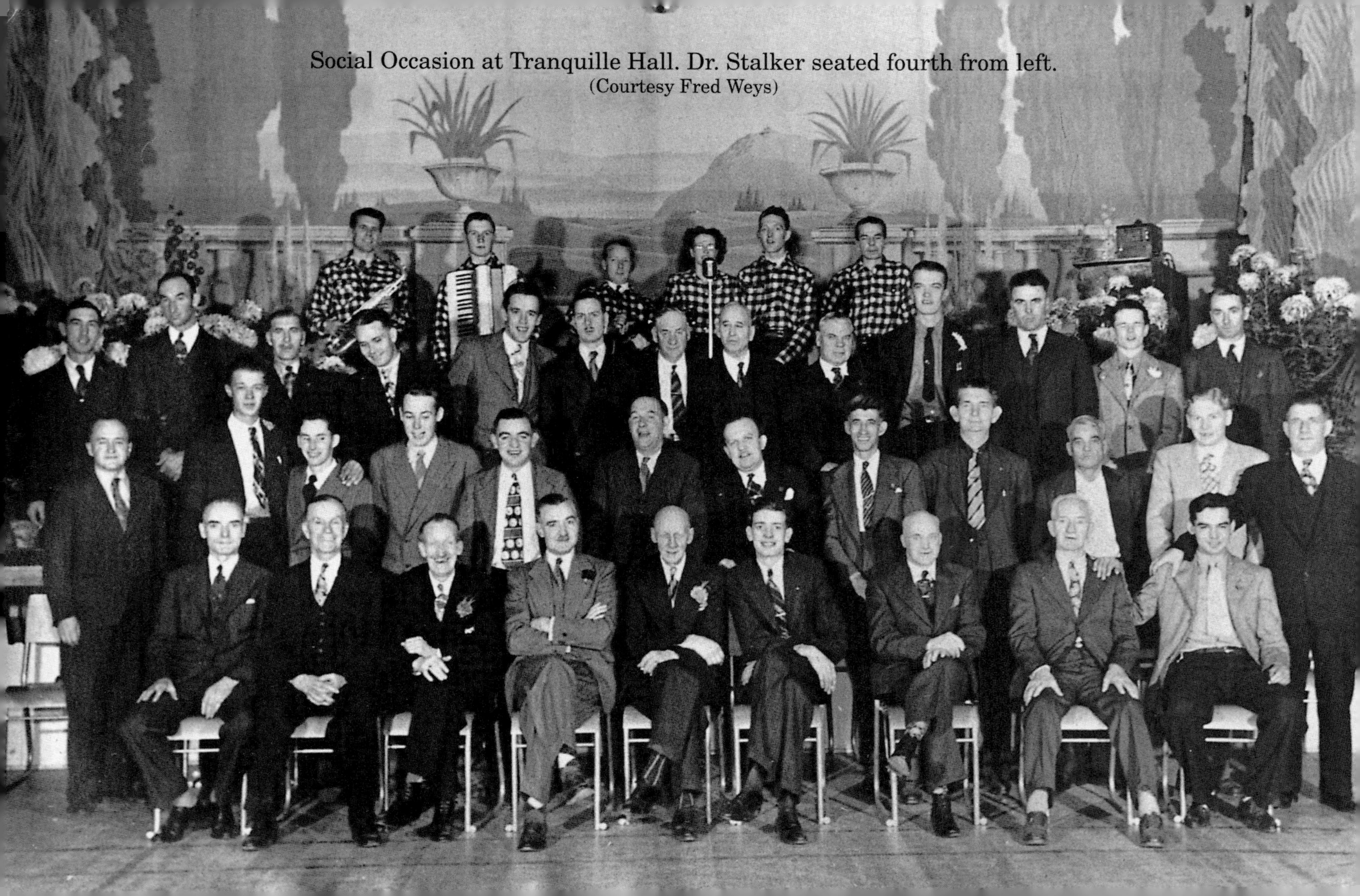

Social Occasion at Tranquille Hall. Dr. Stalker seated fourth from left.
(Courtesy Fred Weys)

The seriousness of the situation finally prodded the government into acting on some of the recommendations concerning accommodation that Stalker had been repeating for years. The ranch boarding house and the old nurses' home were added to in 1948, and the new nurses' home was finally constructed in 1949. Built in the box-like style of architecture favoured at the time, it solved the accommodation problem but looked distinctly odd beside the more gracious older buildings. The administration building was modernized, four new doctors' houses were built, and over a mile of cement sidewalks replaced the familiar cinder paths throughout the grounds.

If modernization was welcomed by staff and patients, there was one occasion when an old system had to be revived to compensate for the failure of a newer one. The flood that struck the Kamloops region in May 1948 did not spare Tranquille. The dam and the water intake installed in 1927 were swept away, and again the institution turned to the old wells. Emergency pumps were rushed from Colony Farm to enable the much-maligned well water to supply the institution once more. The visit of Governor General Viscount Alexander of Tunis went ahead in May as scheduled, but the institution regretted that its reception of a vice-regal party had to coincide with disruptions caused by flood. Within a short time, the water system was repaired and the wells were retired for the last time.

Just as it had in the 1920s, Tranquille benefitted in the late 1940s and early 1950s from the favourable financial position enjoyed by the provincial government. The construction projects of 1948 represent the beginning of a four-year building programme that completely modernized the institution. A comprehensive renovation of the existing medical facilities at Tranquille was recommended by the Tuberculosis Control Branch in 1950 and the government began with extensive renovations to the Infirmary Building. The modernization of the other buildings followed, and by the end of 1952, when the building programme was completed, fifty beds had been added to the institution's capacity. Dr. Stalker eventually pronounced himself pleased with the results, especially with the renovations to the Main Building and with the air conditioning system that had been added to the operating room in the Greaves Building. Just before he concluded his years at the sanatorium, he wrote to an absent colleague: "You would hardly recognize the old place. It really looks like a modern hospital."[15]

However, Tranquille was not the sole beneficiary of additional provincial expenditure on the treatment of tuberculosis. The long planned tuberculosis hospital in the lower mainland finally received the go-ahead in 1950. The contract was let and construction began on property at Cambie Street and 57th Street in South Vancouver. The extensive facility would permit the centralization of tuberculosis care in the lower mainland and eliminate the need for the separate tuberculosis facilities at Jericho Beach, St. Joseph's Oriental Hospital and the City of Vancouver's Isolation Hospital. To be named after the former provincial secretary and minister of health, the Pearson Tuberculosis Hospital was scheduled to open in the spring of 1952.

For the patients, the operation of the newly modernized hospital at Tranquille must have seemed remarkably like the operation of previous years. Every meal, for example, reminded patients of the realities of institutional life. Staff and patient dining rooms were separate, and the crockery clearly indicated further distinctions. Cups and saucers with a blue band were for bed patients only. Those with a green band were used in the patients' cafeteria, those with a red band were for the use of nurses and medical staff, and the plain white dishes were for the non-medical staff. The purpose, of course, was purely hygienic, and any staff member discovered trying to rescue chipped and discarded dishes was in serious trouble. Strict control of the patients' activities was maintained by the medical staff, who insisted upon the separation of the sexes. In other words, all the requirements of rest, rehabilitation, and diet remained, as did the difficulties associated with boredom and recuperation. Some patients took advantage of the occupational therapy classes; others took reading, writing and arithmetic from teachers who were patients themselves. Because of the nature of the shared affliction and because of the length of time many spent at the sanatorium, lasting friendships often developed between patients (as did a few liaisons, despite the best efforts of the vigilant medical staff).

Ambulant patients continued to enjoy the merriment at Christmas and Hallowe'en, adding Easter to the list of opportunities to dress in costume. Even some of those who normally followed the rules looked forward to a Christmas drink, and every year Stalker cautioned patients against this temptation over the radio system. In 1949, for example, he included this statement in his Christmas address:

> One of the most unfortunate and deplorable parts of this season to me is that I sometimes have to deal with individuals who have caused considerable disturbances or trouble by drinking. Let us all spare ourselves any such incidents this year."[16]

Despite the controls, many patients contrived to find ways to break the rules, often taking advantage of the underground tunnel system, sometimes with the connivance of individual support staff.

For bed patients, reading, and listening to the radio remained the chief activities. The magazine *Your Health*, which had replaced *The Tranquillian* in December 1936, was produced in Vancouver and provided little diversion for Tranquille patients. It contained only sparse information about events and personalities at the institution. Gone were the days of "Peter Peeps' Diaries" and poetry competitions. After early 1939, even the popular "Tranquille Notes" column disappeared. However, beginning in the late 1940s, the employees began to produce their *Sanbeam* newsletter and the veterans' voice found expression in their *Fluoroscope*. Both provided detail of interest to Tranquille residents as did the detailed weekly columns submitted by patients to the *Kamloops Sentinel* during 1948.

The separate staff and patients' libraries were extensively used, especially during the daily "rush hour" between 6:30 and 7:30 p.m. The patients' library contained nearly 5,000 volumes by 1944, and recreational reading was seen as an essential part of treatment for patients. Approximately $500 was donated annually by the Canteen towards the purchase of new books. Nearly ninety percent of the bed patients made use of the library, and book repair was part of the occupational therapy programme for a few of the ambulant patients. Several rooms throughout the institution were used, and, for many years, Stalker pressed for the construction of a separate building to centralize the library holdings. Though it was part of the plan for construction in 1948, the central facility was never built. Finally in 1952, the patients' library and the smaller staff library were both housed in the basement of the Infirmary Building. Former patient James Henderson, by this time in receipt of a small salary, continued to act as librarian for the collections.[17]

Yet, the institution was changing, sometimes predictably and sometimes in unanticipated ways. Matron Gladys Currie, described by one of her former nurses as "very, very particular, just like the earlier matrons," resigned in 1946. She was replaced initially by Olive Clancy, and then, in 1948, by Miss Hodgson who could boast a new title—Director of Nursing. The deaths of three former superintendents reminded some of the history of the sanatorium. Dr. Lapp had lost touch with his colleagues in British Columbia, and news of his death in eastern Canada in 1949 was received with surprise. A year later, the first superintendent, Kamloops doctor Robert Irving also passed away, as did Charles Vrooman in Vancouver. The Canadian Tuberculosis Association, holding its fiftieth annual convention at the Hotel Vancouver in May 1950, also gave an indication of changing times. Its programme contained no reference at all to the sanatorium at Tranquille.[18]

After 1945, changes in financial assistance and support organizations also occurred. A rejuvenated British Columbia Tuberculosis Society provided equipment to the sanatorium, as well as welcome moral and financial support in the struggle for a new nurses' home. The federal government (undertaking a nation-wide intervention into health care that would have gladdened the heart of Dr. Fagan) provided the provinces with Dominion Health Grants after 1950. As part of its modernization programme, Tranquille received a sterilizer, photography equipment, and a new pathology laboratory in the first year of the grants. Advances in science and technology were transforming the institution. Refrigeration was introduced just after the war and, for the first time, the institutional need for ice from Kamloops Lake was ended. The air conditioning added to the operating room in 1951 was particularly welcomed by the medical staff.

Most significantly, the introduction of therapeutic drugs radically altered the approach of the medical community in its treatment of the disease. The first effective drug, streptomycin, was developed in the United States and was made available in Canada by 1948. It was soon followed by para-aminosalicylic acid (PAS), which had been developed in Sweden. The tuberculosis bacilli quickly mutated to combat the new drugs, and it was soon necessary to give patients both streptomycin and PAS in order to achieve success. The antimicrobial drugs were joined after 1951 by the even more effective and much cheaper isoniazid (INH). It became apparent that tuberculosis, detected at an early stage, could be controlled by a combination of rest and antimicrobial drugs. Drug treatment and rest made home care more possible for incipient cases and referrals to sanatoria nation-wide began to decline sharply.

Improvements in the condition of patients achieved by drug therapy made surgical intervention possible in many more cases, especially amongst the young. The application of chest surgery increased 400 percent between 1946 and 1950. After 1948, further training of medical staff allowed Tranquille to provide advanced thoracoplastic surgery, intrapleural pneumolysis, thoracoscopy and bronchoscopy. Though the rising population of the province kept the pressure on the ability to accommodate all those afflicted, death rates declined significantly during the late 1940s. As a result of drugs and surgery, death rates for the entire population of the province fell from 57 per 100,000 in 1946 to 27 per 100,000 just four years later.[19]

As the veteran population declined at Tranquille, the numbers of male and female patients had achieved a balance by the mid-1930s that was sustained until the early 1940s. However, by late 1942, the number of male patients was again substantially greater than the number of female patients. That this was occurring even before the arrival of the soldier patients of World War II is significant. It was the beginning of a permanent imbalance in the sex ratios of tubercular patients that was unexpected by medical practitioners. By 1952, the ratio of male to female patients in British Columbia's tuberculosis treatment centres was two to one, and that ratio was much higher in patients over the age of fifty. Half the male patients were over fifty, but only eight percent of women patients were over fifty. Often suffering from advanced stages of the disease, the elderly could benefit from the advantages brought by the new drugs but not from the new surgical techniques. Elderly males in particular became disproportionately represented in the province's institutions and at Tranquille more so than elsewhere. This was partly due to the fact that the declining number of patients requiring just a few months treatment were being kept in the lower mainland, while those in more advanced stages of the disease and requiring more extensive treatment were usually older and were sent to Tranquille.[20]

Changes in the labour force were also occurring. The introduction of the 44-hour workweek in 1947 required alterations in many job categories, particularly those of the non-farm staff. The existence of a branch of the British Columbia Government Employees' Association after World War II also required a period of adjustment in relations between management and employees, though the union had little bargaining power. Ironically, the post-war labour situation saw a return in some respects to the social stratification that Dr. Stalker had so conscientiously sought to eliminate, as both supervisory staff and regular employees adjusted to the new arrangements. One consequence of this new relationship was the formation of a full-time regular fire department at Tranquille. Under department chief "Chuck" Sealy, fire drills became more frequent, but it would be the good fortune of the new regular fire department that it would never be required to fight a real fire. Over the years, members of the department were known to both boast and lament that they were never called upon to put their skills to a genuine test.

Significant changes also took place at the senior administrative level. By September 1950, Mary Rowles had become the new director of nursing, bringing to the position ability that was widely acknowledged. Less than two years later, she would provide much of the continuity in administration as the institution prepared to say farewell to Dr. Stalker. For just the second time in its thirty years as a provincially-run institution, the Tranquille Sanatorium was to have a new medical superintendent. During Stalker's fifteen years in charge, Tranquille had become a sanatorium widely regarded as the best in Canada, and it was the general opinion of both patients and staff that Stalker's personal reputation matched that of the institution. His resignation took effect 31 December 1951, and he was transferred to Vancouver. He was to become the first medical superintendent of the Pearson Hospital which, after nearly twenty years of discussion and planning, finally opened in May 1952.

Chapter Notes

1 British Columbia Archives and Records Service (BCARS), GR 108, box 6, file 3, Stalker to G.F. Kincade, 22 November 1951.
2 BCARS, GR 108, box 1, file 2, Madge Farmer to Stalker, 21 March 1940.
3 BCARS, GR 497, box 8, file 7; GR 496, box 23, file 12.
4 BCARS, GR 497, box 8, file 7.
5 BCARS, GR 108, box 5, file 5, Stalker to Hatfield, 16 October 1940.
6 The Cooney orchard was uprooted towards the end of the 1940s. All that remained of the Cooney experience was the family cemetery, which the government promised to tend in perpetuity.
7 *Victoria Daily Colonist*, 25 October 1944, p. 11.
8 BCARS, GR 497, box 8, file 7; GR 496, box 51, file 5.
9 BCARS, GR 496, box 51, file 4; *Vancouver Sun*, 1 June 1940, p. 17; *Kamloops Sentinel*, 7 November 1940, p. 10.
10 *Kamloops Sentinel*, 8 September 1943, p. 1; Les King interview, 13 December 1998.
11 Patricia Koretchuk, David Caldow memoir; *Kamloops Sentinel*, 29 March 1944, p. 1; Gerry Rositch interview, 8 December 1998.
12 *Vancouver Province*, 22 November 1944, p. 11.
13 *Vancouver News-Herald*, 21 June 1946, p. 1; *Victoria Daily Times*, 22 June 1946, p. 11; British Columbia *Sessional Papers* 1948, volume 1, First Report of the Department of Health and Welfare, p. J 73.
14 BCARS, GR 129, box 7, file 2.
15 BCARS, GR 108, box 6, file 3, Stalker to W.G. Trapp, 24 September 1951.
16 BCARS, GR 108, box 6, file 3.
17 BCARS, GR 108, box 4, file 4.
18 National Archives of Canada, MG 28 I 75, Records of the Canadian Tuberculosis Association, volume 1, file 2.
19 British Columbia *Sessional Papers* 1948-1953, Reports of the Department of Health and Welfare and the Division of Tuberculosis Control.
20 British Columbia *Sessional Papers* 1953-54 volume 1, Report of the Division of Tuberculosis Control, p. F15; British Columbia *Sessional Papers* 1956, Report of the Division of Tuberculosis Control, p. D15.

"A Whole Little City by Itself" The Final Years

The opening of the Pearson Hospital ushered in a new era of tuberculosis care in British Columbia. The first patients admitted to the new institution were indicative of that new era: nine Japanese internees who previously had been treated in the segregated tuberculosis hospital at New Denver.[1] The Pearson Hospital provided the lower mainland with a large, centralized treatment facility for tuberculosis for the first time, and elimination of some of the smaller centres in Vancouver was expected. All beds were quickly filled, and with the capacity of the new facility added to the increased capacity at Tranquille, the provincial waiting list was sharply reduced. It was perhaps inevitable that the new hospital, located where the majority of the tubercular patients of the province actually lived, would also lead to a further decline in the significance of the Tranquille Sanatorium. It was certainly not anticipated that the institution near Kamloops would suffer a total eclipse, and that its closure would occur before the decade was over.

Replacing Stalker as medical superintendent at Tranquille was Dr. Frederick Oren Roswell Garner. For a short period during the mid-1930s, Garner (who preferred the nickname "Roscoe") had provided summer relief for the medical staff at Tranquille. At the end of 1936, he entered private practice in Vancouver, and, from 1946, had been the medical superintendent of the Victoria Unit of the Tuberculosis Branch. He took over at the Tranquille Unit just as the renovation of the Main Building and the Infirmary was finally completed, increasing the capacity of the sanatorium to 410 beds. With patient and employee numbers combined, the population at Tranquille was in excess of six hundred people.

Upon Dr. Garner's arrival, one of Dr. Lapp's perennial recommendations was finally implemented: an administrative assistant was added to the staff of the sanatorium in order to allow the medical superintendent to focus more completely upon medical matters. In fact, each previous superintendent had complained that too much of his time was taken by the requirements of administration. Dr. Garner took charge of the facility at its peak capacity, and enjoyed the advantage over his predecessors of being able to delegate many of the tasks involved in the day-to-day running of the institution. Though he would face administrative tasks not contemplated at the time of his appointment, Garner probably did not expect to be the first and only medical superintendent at Tranquille untroubled by waiting lists.

The year 1952 was a time of political confusion for British Columbia, but by year's end, the province had a new government: W.A.C. Bennett's Social Credit Party. The new administration was immediately subjected to the same pressures as its predecessors concerning considerations of patronage. For example, Health Minister Eric Martin soon received a letter from a patient at Tranquille demanding a complete overhaul of hospital administration. Writing as "a supporter of Social Credit and a taxpayer," the letter writer also complained about the persistent power outages and insisted that the problem of flies at Tranquille be dealt with.[2] Perhaps because the administration of the institution had been completely overhauled just a few months earlier, or perhaps because an informal investigation found no unacceptable political partisanship, the new government was initially able to resist pressure to return to the pre-war system of political appointments at Tranquille. Garner continued as medical superintendent and Mary Rowles remained as director of nursing. Farm manager David Caldow was transferred to Colony Farm at the end of 1953, but the transfer was not politically motivated. His successor, thirty-two-year-old Les King, had worked at Tranquille as a ranch hand from 1941 until 1946 when a World War II veteran returned to reclaim his position. King had then been transferred to Essondale, returning to Tranquille as farm manager in early 1954.

Upon his return, King noted one significant change. The teams of workhorses were gone. Only saddle horses remained as the farm had become almost completely mechanized. Otherwise, the operation of the Tranquille complex followed patterns that were well established by the 1940s. The farm increased its small beef herd somewhat in the 1950s, but kept its focus on dairy production. The sixty-five head of registered Holstein cattle needed milking three times daily, providing all the dairy requirements of the sanatorium, as well as a surplus for sale. The piggery and the cannery also continued to provide a substantial proportion of the institution's food needs. At least a dozen Yorkshire hogs and two cows were slaughtered by abattoir workers every week. A dozen beehives provided as much as eight hundred pounds of honey annually. Though much of the fruit canned at Tranquille was not produced by the small orchard there, the vegetable gardens provided more than the sanatorium required. The surplus went to correctional facilities in the Kamloops area, the Provincial Old Men's Home, and Essondale.

The Dominion Health Grants added materially to the maintenance of modern equipment throughout the decade. The gardens continued to attract visitors, and dignitaries continued to provide an official presence: visits are recorded by Lieutenant Governor Clarence Wallace in August 1952 and Governor General Vincent Massey in May 1953. Performing groups continued to include Tranquille in their schedules: Chief Dan George and his Burrard Indian Orchestra and Dancers performed on the lawns for a large audience in August 1957. Veterans continued to receive donations from their former comrades-in-arms: branches of the Canadian Legion provided money, cigarettes, and the patients' first television set.[3]

In many respects, Garner was faced with the same problems that had perplexed earlier superintendents: among them, a shortage of nurses, sewage concerns, and the disregard for sanatorium regulations shown by some patients. The difficulty in retaining a full complement of competent nurses had presented a problem for the Tranquille Sanatorium since the days of the First World War. Though part of a province-wide problem, the shortage at Tranquille was compounded by the general opinion in British Columbia at the time that any community outside the lower mainland was properly considered isolated. Apart from sanatorium nurses resident in Kamloops (though they, too, often left for jobs at the Royal Inland Hospital), the province's nurses in the 1950s continued the patterns of their predecessors by preferring employment elsewhere.

The issue of sewage disposal, a problem for the sanatorium since 1907, again demanded attention in early 1955. The South Central Health Unit in Kamloops called for the erection of warning signs close to where the sewage from the sanatorium was discharged into Kamloops Lake. Though the Health Unit felt there was "no actual danger to health because of the large dilution factor," they wanted the upper part of the lake declared "unfit for recreational purposes." After a year of inaction on the issue, the Kamloops Rod and Gun Club and the Kamloops Fish and Game Protective Association added their voices to the call for action on the "deplorable situation" of sewage treatment at Tranquille. The government responded by installing a three-acre stabilization pond on the old horse meadow by the lake shore in March 1957. However, it did not operate satisfactorily due to faulty construction.[4]

Dr. Garner fought the same battle against the use of alcohol as had all previous superintendents. Visitors, especially those seeing "suspect" patients, were often asked by head nurses or the director of nursing to reveal the contents of purses and packages. A Kamloops taxi driver was convicted in 1955 of bootlegging, and two male employees were under suspicion of supplying alcohol to patients. The problem was complicated inadvertently by Kamloops' new Social Credit MLA. Without consulting the hospital administration, Phil Gaglardi arranged with the minister of health to permit the Kinsmen to hold their annual convention at the sanatorium in 1957. The delegates behaved as they would have done at any of their conventions elsewhere, but the evident consumption of alcohol presented difficulties for Dr. Garner and his staff. G.F. Kincade, Director of the Division of Tuberculosis Control, urged the minister of health to turn down a subsequent request from the Independent Order of Odd Fellows to use the sanatorium facilities for their convention. He noted his department's displeasure at the decision concerning the Kinsmen. The Kinsmen convention of 1957 was the only such event ever to be held at the sanatorium.[5]

One decision taken by the Social Credit government certainly presented difficulties at Tranquille. Previously, with the shortage of beds throughout the province, the minister of health rarely used his authority to force reluctant patients to take treatment. With beds becoming more readily available, Health Minister Eric Martin in 1953 designated one tubercular male as a menace to public health and ordered him into a care facility. He did the same in three cases in 1954, nine times in 1955 and four times in 1956. Most of the recalcitrant patients were sent to Tranquille because of the isolation of the sanatorium and because the Tranquille Unit was the only tuberculosis facility in the province containing a few rooms that could be secured if necessary. Though there were never more than seven such patients at Tranquille at a time, their numbers often included Oakalla prisoners, distinctly unhappy at having been transferred to the sanatorium against their will. In 1956, two such patients "were confined in a restraining area" because they would not cooperate, and because they had "shown a defiance of the committal order," and had "left the sanatorium without permission." Surprisingly, few employees were made aware of the special character of these patients. Members of the fire department were given the responsibility of keeping the recalcitrant patients under surveillance. The lock-up rooms were rarely used, and no serious incidents are recorded.[6]

Another group of reluctant patients was formed by Hungarian refugees. Admitted to Canada after the unsuccessful uprising in Budapest in 1956, at least a dozen of those who came to British Columbia were found to have tuberculosis. They were sent to Tranquille, where a member of the nursing staff who spoke Hungarian acted as a translator. Many were displeased that they were required to spend time at the sanatorium, but most were discharged after only a short stay.

Death rates from tuberculosis continued their dramatic decline, both nationally and provincially. British Columbia's death rate of 11.5 per 100,000 population in 1953 contrasted sharply with the death rate of 57.4 per 100,000 in 1947. The application of drugs, surgical intervention, and preventative measures combined to achieve this result. The BCG (Bacillus of Calmette and Guérin) vaccine was administered widely amongst Natives, nurses, and hospital workers and was found effective approximately 80 percent of the time for those who had been exposed to tuberculosis. In 1953, the Report of the Division of Tuberculosis Control stated directly for the first time that tuberculosis "can now be cured."[7]

New dimensions to treatment at Tranquille were provided by the increased use of drugs and by the application of more extensive surgical intervention. With the arrival of Dr. William McLaren in 1952, the sanatorium acquired the services of a full-time surgeon for the first time in its history. Surgery was increasingly recommended for patients whose condition would not fully respond to the use of what were, by this time, referred to as the "miracle drugs": streptomycin, INH and PAS. With the diminishing pressure of waiting lists, patients were subject to less pressure to leave before their medical conditions permitted. By the end of 1953, though all of the 800 tuberculosis beds available in British Columbia were occupied, the waiting list had virtually disappeared. The provincial pattern matched that in the rest of the country, in the United States and in Western Europe. Death rates from tuberculosis were falling rapidly. Sanatoria in Germany, Switzerland, and Sweden began to close. Edward Trudeau's famous sanatorium at Saranac closed its doors in 1954.

In most respects, however, the day to day operation of the institution at Tranquille remained as it had for decades. The shortage of nurses continued, usually receiving a note of concern in the annual reports of the Tuberculosis Division. The patients generally continued to acquiesce in the traditional regime of rest and inactivity. A few, however, resisted by receiving "unauthorized" guests at unorthodox times, escaping for a quick cigarette, or lamenting that a long-anticipated bottle of liquor had been discovered by a nurse in the purse of a visitor. The employees living in the men's home, the maids' home and the ranch house continued to grumble about regular visits from the matron to ensure that the institution's required standards of hygiene were being maintained. Presumably, the living quarters of the doctors and nurses needed no such matronly tours of inspection.

If living conditions remained essentially the same after the late 1940s, working conditions certainly changed. The introduction of the forty-hour workweek for all provincial employees early in 1955 presented the same difficulties for administration as had the reductions of working hours in 1938, 1942, and 1947. Approximately twenty new employees were required (most of them nurses, nurses' aides and ward assistants), and assignments in many job categories were altered. The institution's payroll rose by nearly $4,000 per month.

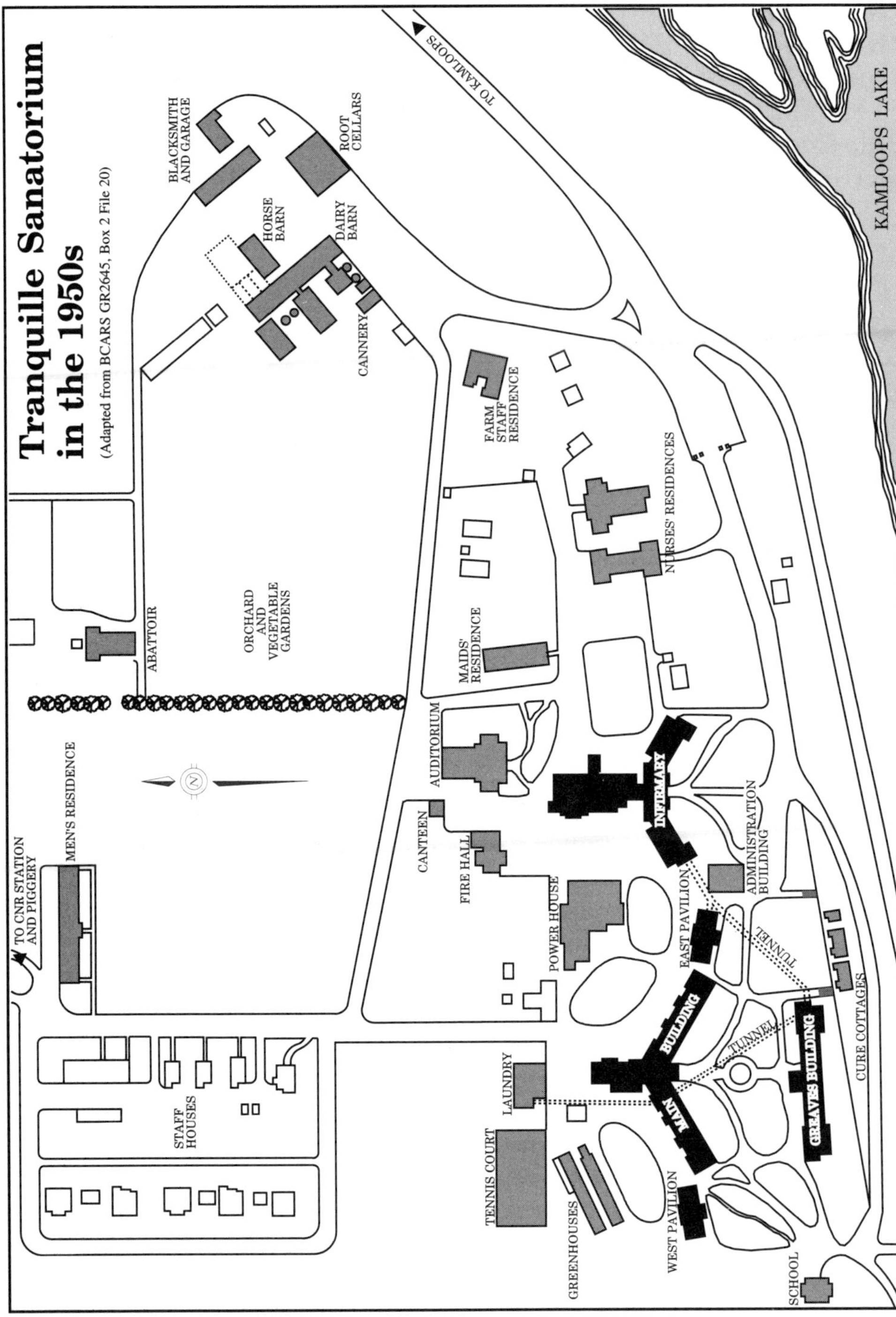

Tranquille Sanatorium in the 1950s
(Adapted from BCARS GR2645, Box 2 File 20)
BLACKSMITH AND GARAGE
ROOT CELLARS
TO KAMLOOPS
HORSE BARN
DAIRY BARN
CANNERY
KAMLOOPS LAKE
FARM STAFF RESIDENCE
NURSES' RESIDENCES
ORCHARD AND VEGETABLE GARDENS
ABATTOIR
MAIDS' RESIDENCE
AUDITORIUM
INFIRMARY
ADMINISTRATION BUILDING
MEN'S RESIDENCE
TO CNR STATION AND PIGGERY
CANTEEN
FIRE HALL
POWER HOUSE
EAST PAVILION
TUNNEL
BUILDING
MAIN
TUNNEL
GREAVES BUILDING
CURE COTTAGES
STAFF HOUSES
LAUNDRY
TENNIS COURT
GREENHOUSES
WEST PAVILION
SCHOOL

Some savings were achieved by closing the kitchen at the ranch house in May 1955. Farm workers subsequently took their meals with other employees in the staff cafeteria in the Service Building.[8]

Kamloops and Closure

The prospect of closing the sanatorium generated within the community of Kamloops a controversy of considerable magnitude. Kamloops was as reluctant to see the institution close in the 1950s as it had been to see it open in 1907. The loss of a payroll of approximately $1 million would be a serious blow to the local economy. Rumours about closure began to circulate as early as 1954. In reply to a formal enquiry, Health Minister Eric Martin wrote to Kamloops Mayor J.E. Fitzwater in August 1954 to assure him the government did not intend to close any of the buildings at Tranquille. However, as patient numbers declined, circumstances changed rapidly. The Main Building was the first to be closed early in 1956 and was joined by the East Pavilion by the end of the year. The seriousness of the situation was suddenly brought home to most Kamloops residents by a newspaper report. The *Kamloops Sentinel*, following the Vancouver newspapers, reported on 31 October 1956 that the site was being considered for use as a federal penitentiary. There followed a flurry of telegrams to Ottawa and Victoria opposing the idea from city council, the Kamloops and District Board of Trade, and the South Central Union Board of Health. The rumour proved to be false, but with the provincial death rate less than eight per 100,000 by 1956, it was obvious that the closing of the Tranquille Sanatorium could not be far off.

For several months, as they awaited an official announcement, people in Kamloops debated the merits of various proposals to convert the institution. Should it become an agricultural college or a retirement home, a hospital for the chronically or mentally ill, an art college or a vocational school? By May 1957, the last of Victoria's tuberculosis patients was transferred to Vancouver as treatment was rapidly becoming centralized at the Willow Chest Clinic and the Pearson Tuberculosis Hospital. At Tranquille, chest surgery was eliminated in March 1957, and, just after the closure of a second floor of the Greaves Building in July, employees were officially advised that the institution would close completely within a year. By this time, Dr.

McLaren had entered private practice in Kamloops and Dr. Gee had elected to retire in Vancouver. At the end of August, as the government made public its intention to close the facility, Mary Rowles left Tranquille to become the director of nursing at the Royal Inland Hospital. Eva Moody became matron. She would be the last. One Kamloops council member expressed the fear that Tranquille was about to become a "white elephant".[9]

Still no announcement came and, in September 1957, even local government supporters expressed their annoyance at the lack of progress on the issue. A few days later, Eric Martin advised the board of Royal Inland Hospital that it could proceed with plans to build a ward for chronic care. Clearly, the possibility of Tranquille becoming a chronic care hospital had been removed from the table, but another winter passed without decision about the future of the facility. In February 1958, Martin announced the facility would close by the end of the year. In March, he travelled to Kamloops to speak at an election meeting in support of the local Social Credit candidate in the federal election. The health minister found the gathering well attended, largely by Tranquille employees demanding information and answers. Martin returned to Victoria convinced that the community of Kamloops was "seething" over the issue of Tranquille's future.[10]

Local MLA and Minister of Highways Phil Gaglardi privately told individual sanatorium employees they had no cause to worry. Letters from nurses and former patients in support of keeping the facility open began to appear in the *Kamloops Sentinel*. The Kamloops Board of Trade formally protested the closure on 1 May, urging that the government use the facility for "mental defectives." The Board of Trade also sponsored a petition that garnered 1,700 signatures, while more than a hundred business owners sent telegrams to Premier W.A.C. Bennett urging the continuance of the facility in one form or another. In June, the Kamloops School Board's proposal for use of the facility as a vocational college was endorsed by the British Columbia School Trustees' Association.

Finally, on 10 June, Gaglardi issued an official statement that the buildings would be used by the government "for some purpose," that most employees would be able to keep their jobs, and that a government committee was examining the options. The *Sentinel* broke its editorial silence on the closure by supporting the Board of Trade proposal that Tranquille become a home for "mental defectives of the non-dangerous variety." As remaining patients continued to be transferred to Vancouver's Pearson Hospital and as rumours continued to circulate, the community waited for further details of the government's intentions. Transfers of individual employees also continued, and the school board announced that declining student enrolment required the closure of the Tranquille School at the end of June.

The local uproar began to attract attention in the lower mainland. One letter in the *Vancouver Sun* demanded to know why columnists Simma Holt and Jack Scott had not commented upon the issue. The challenge was taken up by another *Sun* writer, Elmore Philpott, who visited Tranquille in early June "to find out what the fuss and fury was all about." What he found, evidently to his surprise, was "a whole little city in itself." He noted that the hospital, with its attendant fire hall, power plant, laundry and farm, could treat not just tuberculosis patients, but patients of any description. He noted it would be very expensive to start up again if it were allowed to close, and concluded "every intelligent man, woman and child in Kamloops was determined not to let this great social crime come to pass."[11]

Losing patience at the end of June, the Kamloops Board of Trade demanded to know just who was on the government committee and what it was doing. The dispute with Gaglardi raged throughout the month of July. Gaglardi claimed he was now head of the probe examining future use, while the Board of Trade accused Bennett, Gaglardi, and Health Minister Martin of giving it the run-around on the question. It concluded that Gaglardi's committee was either "non-existent or lacking sufficient direction to reach a decision." Responding to "keep the record straight," Gaglardi claimed he had never heard from the Board of Trade on the matter and said it appeared that somebody was "trying to play a game." He avoided mention of any committee. Clearly, the sanatorium had again become a political football.[12]

As late as the end of August, Eric Martin suggested to the British Columbia Hospital Association that the facility would be appropriately used as an extended care hospital for the aged. However, on 2 September, Gaglardi personally telephoned the *Kamloops Sentinel* to advise that an announcement was about to be made. Tranquille was to be used as a home for "mentally defective" adults between twenty and forty years old who were not a risk to the community. The new patients would be transferred from overcrowded facilities at Woodlands and Essondale in the lower mainland. The campaign run by the Kamloops Board of Trade and the *Sentinel* had succeeded.

The announcement by Eric Martin on 3 September 1958 meant political hesitation was over and legal difficulties had been overcome. By law, the facility at Tranquille could be used only for the treatment of tuberculosis. The proposal to operate a home for the mentally handicapped, therefore, was technically contrary to the terms of the government takeover of 1921. However, the British Columbia Tuberculosis Society, the legal successor to the British Columbia Anti-Tuberculosis Society, raised no objections to the proposal. The society wanted the buildings at Tranquille put to humanitarian use and believed that the defeat of tuberculosis was assured. The government was thereby released from what could have become awkward obligations and proceeded with its plans to re-open under the Department of Mental Health.[13]

Politically triumphant and at peace with the Kamloops Board of Trade, Gaglardi almost immediately found himself embroiled in controversy with the sanatorium employees. On 29 August, employees were formally advised that the institution would close on 4 October. The appointment of Dr. Garner as the new medical superintendent at Pearson Hospital was announced, and the transfers of other doctors and nurses were confirmed. Most of the remaining eight-nine employees, however, were still wondering what their fate was to be. With no assurances of employment after 4 October and ineligible for unemployment insurance as employees of the provincial government, they held a meeting at the Tranquille recreation hall on 21 September. The meeting appointed a delegation to meet with Gaglardi and asked for assistance from their union, the British Columbia Government Employees Association. Over the next few days, Gaglardi pointed out that, though the Board of Trade had "roused the citizens" to demand a mental institution, no one should expect the transition to be completely without difficulties. He assured BCGEA members that the first mental patients would arrive "sometime in October," but temporary layoffs were unavoidable until then.[14] He told the employees the institution would be running again within six weeks, but local BCGEA president W.H. Paterson and provincial general-secretary Ed O'Connor noted there were no government plans to support such optimism. They were right. The first mental health patients would not arrive at Tranquille until July 1959.

The process created a bitterness that lingered in Kamloops for many years. It was an unfortunate and apparently unnecessary legacy. The difficult period of adjustment required by the closing of the institution was complicated by Gaglardi's apparent desire to promise all things to all people and his tendency to speak even when it was apparent he did not have the facts. Undoubtedly, he was in a difficult position. If the opening of the institution in 1907 had been achieved with an air of desperation and confusion, the closure bore all the same characteristics. The government seemed uncertain how to proceed. Undecided about what to do with the facility, it left Gaglardi to complicate matters with a confusion of policies and possibilities as the months rolled by.

Final Days

All of the attention received by the political posturing deflected attention from the sanatorium as it quietly wrapped up its operation of more than fifty years. If a commemoration of the fiftieth anniversary of the operation of the Tranquille Sanatorium occurred in November 1957, it was not noted in newspapers and government records. Perhaps by that time, with the closure imminent, few were inclined to celebrate. Patient numbers by January 1958 had been reduced to just over one hundred, and transfers to Vancouver were occurring regularly. The equipment purchased for Tranquille through the Dominion Health Grants was moved to the Royal Inland Hospital. Most of the nearly 7,000 volumes in the patients' library were made available to the Pearson Tuberculosis Hospital in Vancouver. The final several weeks were hectic ones at the institution, with Dr. Garner advising the provincial secretary on one occasion that he could not report on arrangements because events were "moving too fast to record."

By the end of July, fewer than forty patients were receiving treatment at Tranquille. The ten remaining female patients expressed their reluctance to go to Vancouver, but several of them nevertheless were among the party of eighteen placed on a special CNR car at Tranquille station on 19 August. To remain at Tranquille was no longer an option. By mid-September, only one ward—located in the Greaves Building containing fifteen elderly male and four female patients—was still operating. For reasons of economy, even the strict separation of the sexes had evidently been abandoned for the final few days. The last of the patients left Tranquille on the evening of 23 September, catching the night train to Vancouver.[15]

October third, a beautiful autumn day, was the final day of work for maids, kitchen help and orderlies. The farm staff, the fire department and public works employees were all advised a few days earlier that they would stay on for maintenance and protection. A reporter for the *Sentinel* spent that last day at Tranquille. He wrote that the beds in the empty wards were all stripped of their white tailored sheets. What seemed like miles of corridors were silent and empty. He noted the signs commanding visitors to keep off the well-kept lawns had no fear of contradiction.[16] Accompanying his article was a poignant photograph of the last few staff members walking through the main gate to catch the last bus to Kamloops. The departure through the gate of the housekeepers and cleaners, accompanied by nurses Evelyn Connolly and Jean Woodbury, brought to a conclusion the work that Dr. Fagan and the British Columbia Anti-Tuberculosis Society had begun.

For more than fifty years, doctors, nurses, and support staff had been engaged in the treatment and care of thousands of victims of what once had been the most deadly disease in the province of British Columbia. Their services at Tranquille were no longer required.

Chapter Notes

1 British Columbia Lung Association Archives, box 1, Esther Paulson, "TB Nursing 1908-1968."
2 British Columbia Archives and Records Service (BCARS), GR 129, box 18, Tranquille Sanatorium.
3 BCARS, GR 129, box 36, file 13, *The Fluoroscope*, July/August 1957.
4 BCARS, GR 129, box 32, file 4; *Kamloops Sentinel*, 7 May 1957, p. 10.
5 BCARS, GR 129, box 36, file 13.
6 British Columbia *Sessional Papers* 1956, 1957, 1958, Reports of the Tuberculosis Division 1954, 1955, 1956.
7 British Columbia *Sessional Papers* 1955, Report of the Division of Tuberculosis Control, p. D13.
8 BCARS, GR 129, box 28, file 19.
9 *Kamloops Sentinel*, 29 August 1957, p. 3.
10 *Kamloops Sentinel,* 28 March 1958, p. 1.
11 *Vancouver Sun*, 14 June 1958, p. 4.
12 *Kamloops Sentinel*, 29 July 1958, p. 1; 30 July 1958, pp. 1-2.
13 British Columbia Lung Association Archives, box 1.
14 *Kamloops Sentinel*, 24 September 1958, p. 1; 29 September 1958, p. 3.
15 BCARS, GR 129, box 40, file 2.
16 *Kamloops Sentinel*, 4 October 1958, p. 1, John Picton, "Tranquille - Memories and a Question Mark."

Proud History, Awkward Legacy

The buildings were put to good use for many years after 1958. They were thoroughly renovated as the site was converted to a facility for the educable mentally retarded. With a change in government policy, the institution closed for a second time in 1984. The property sat unused for many years and was subjected to much vandalism, though several families continued to rent houses from the government. Proposals and suggestions for utilization of the facility were again widely considered, as nearly all the same suggestions of the late 1950s resurfaced: a veterinarian or agricultural college, a resort, a working farm, a correctional centre. Finally, in 1991, the property was purchased by Giovanni Camporese of A&A Foods in Vancouver for just $8 million, with the provincial government holding the mortgage. He announced grand plans to establish a destination resort.

Then, to the annoyance of nearly everyone locally, Camporese renamed the property Padova City after his own birthplace in Italy. He did not act on his development plans and, over the next few years, the property was allowed to deteriorate. He stopped making mortgage and tax payments in 1995. Just as a reluctant William and Jane Fortune had repossessed the property in the 1890s, a distinctly reluctant provincial government finally repossessed the property in 1998 and placed it on the market once more. No acceptable offers to purchase were received, so the city of Kamloops, owed more than a million dollars in taxes on the property, became the new owner.

Those who declared that the sanatorium at Tranquille would stand as "a lasting monument" both to Dr. Fagan and to the antituberculosis movement would be saddened to see the site today. The sadness would not derive from the knowledge that the old enemy apparently had been defeated. The "miracle of the empty beds," as Doctor W.G. Wherrett so aptly described the victory of medical science, would have been profoundly pleasing to them all. Their sadness would result instead from the appearance of the dilapidated sanatorium buildings, which project not an image of triumph, but rather a sense of ruin and abandonment.

Whatever plans for the future may emerge, the next owner will first have to decide how to cope with the remnants of the past. Just after the government takeover in 1921, one newspaper reporter described the tuberculosis institution as a "fine pile o' buildings." Many observers today would use the phrase without the adjective. The four remaining hospital buildings—Main, East Pavilion, West Pavilion, and even Greaves—have lost their grandeur. Renovations to the structures' exteriors since the early 1940s, such as the removal of balconies from the Main Building and the addition of fire escapes, damaged the pleasing architectural appearance of the institution. The site today presents an impression of random and makeshift construction. The support buildings, built at different times in different styles, and subject to much alteration in design and function over the years, add to this impression. The fine old nurses' home was demolished in the mid-1960s, leaving only a large patch of empty ground beside the box-like new nurses' home of 1949. As part of a reconstruction of the Service Building at the same time, Charles Bentall's Infirmary was also demolished. A long grey plywood covering conceals the tunnels that still run underground to the other buildings. The front road entrance, no longer accessible by car, seems to lead only to a confusing, decrepit and somehow forbidding pile of buildings. Those familiar with the institution during its working life are distressed at the sight of it today.

For the third time, suggestions about the possible use of the property are being discussed. Many of the same questions are being asked. Would Tranquille be viable as an agricultural or veterinary college, as a federal penitentiary, as a hospital of some sort? However, some suggestions seem less practical than they once were. The viability of the property as a resort is compromised by the proximity of the Weyerhaeuser pulp mill and by the fiasco of the Camporese years, which hastened the deterioration of the buildings. Newer suggestions include using the property as a permanent site for movie or television productions of the thriller or horror variety, as a halfway house for convicts, or as a fire-fighting training facility. Interestingly, a portion of the property at Gravenhurst in Ontario, where the first sanatorium in Canada was established by the National Sanitarium Association over a century ago, has been used as a provincial training facility for fire fighters since 1957. Most former sanatoria throughout Canada have been successfully converted to other uses. Perhaps, by the time this history is published, the fate of Tranquille will have been decided. Perhaps the renovation or, more likely, the demolition of the buildings will have begun.

The attitude of Kamloops towards the institution at Tranquille at the end of the century has reverted to mirror what it was at the beginning of the century. Essentially, the old property is seen as an economic liability to the city and as a health threat. The city administrator has stated that the City of Kamloops has "no wish to take over the site, its $500,000 environmental cleanup cost, demolition costs and $180,000 annual upkeep." With concerns about water supply, sewage treatment, land contamination, the presence of asbestos, tax and liability issues, as well as uncertainty about future use, the City of Kamloops seems to wish the institution simply did not exist. The issues facing the current council are just as complex as those facing Mayor Michel in 1904. However, while the council and business establishment of the early century did not want a sanatorium in their future, the present council and community must acknowledge that they had one in their past.

The Tranquille Sanatorium played an integral part in the economic, social and political history of Kamloops for more than fifty years, though it may have left an awkward legacy. Perhaps an indication of both the history and the legacy was the widespread distaste expressed by residents of Kamloops at the announcement that the location was to be renamed in 1991. Rumours about the site, always a potent factor in Kamloops historically, still circulate regularly. Amongst the younger population, there exist firm convictions that Tranquille was an asylum for the insane, that ghosts of an evil disposition inhabit the buildings, that abuse of patients was widespread at the institution. Amongst the older population, rumours of a pending sale to usually wealthy and distant buyers gain ready credence. Most of the personal memories held by local people now concern only the operation under the auspices of the Department of Mental Health. The days of tuberculosis treatment seem distant.

With the demolition of the buildings at Tranquille apparently imminent, it should be recognized how much will be lost. In 1914, upon the death of Dr. Fagan, the Anti-Tuberculosis Society took the position that no memorial other than the sanatorium would be required to honour the memory of the man whose efforts had created the institution. The society itself has had no acknowledgement of the work it did in health care and philanthropy. At the Tranquille site, the deserted buildings serve to motivate the curious to ask questions about their history. They find the answers lead back to the beginning of the century, to the antituberculosis movement, to controversies. In addition to the private operation, millions of provincial tax dollars and years of government effort in health care are represented by the silent structures. So, too, are the legacies of G.B. Greaves, of the many smaller private bequests, and of the work of medical and non-medical staff employed at Tranquille over nearly eighty years.

This book was undertaken to record at least a portion of that legacy. What began as an exercise in local history soon expanded to include necessary elements of the provincial, national and international story. Nevertheless, the intention remained to keep the institution at Tranquille as the study's focus. The sanatorium at Tranquille clearly had a life of its own. Everyone who was kind enough to share memories and impressions of Tranquille mentioned that it was a very special place indeed. Those who attended school there, those who worked there, and even those who were patients there all agree about that. Yet, the atmosphere of a tuberculosis sanatorium is particularly difficult to explain. Amongst the many letters the institution received over the years from appreciative patients is one that says simply: "I was far happier at Tranquille than I expected to be." It is a significant statement. Perhaps, in considering it, even those of us fortunate enough never to have been its patients can derive some understanding of the experience of life in the sanatorium at Tranquille.

A Note on Sources

Readers interested in pursuing the topic further have a wide range of secondary literature and primary sources available to them.

The fight against tuberculosis is discussed by Nobel Prize winner Selman Waksman, *The Conquest of Tuberculosis* (Berkeley, 1966), and by René and Jean Dubos, *The White Plague* (Toronto, 1952). The story of Trudeau's sanatorium and its famous patients is superbly told by Robert Taylor, *Saranac: America's Magic Mountain* (Boston, 1986). For a philosophical look at the disease, see Susan Sontag, *Illness as Metaphor* (New York, 1978). An excellent historical analysis is provided by Linda Bryder, *Below the Magic Mountain: A Social History of Tuberculosis in Twentieth Century Britain* (Oxford, 1988). The differing Canadian and American responses to the disease are examined by Georgina Feldberg, *Disease and Class: Tuberculosis and the Shaping of Modern North American Society* (New Brunswick, New Jersey, 1995). The history of tuberculosis is receiving renewed attention as the late-century threat increases. Frank Ryan's splendid *The Forgotten Plague* (Boston, 1992) provides a historical discussion and a consideration of the current situation.

The Canadian story is told by G.J. Wherrett, *The Miracle of the Empty Beds: A History of Tuberculosis in Canada* (Toronto, 1977) and by Edward. A. Allen's forthcoming "Tuberculosis: A History of the Disease in Canada" in the *Canadian Medical Journal*. Surgical intervention is considered by Norman C. Delarue, *Thoracic Surgery in Canada* (Toronto, 1989). The veterans' story is analysed by Desmond Morton and Glenn Wright, *Winning The Second Battle: Canadian Veterans and the Return to Civilian Life 1915-1930* (Toronto, 1987). J.T.H. Connor, *A Heritage of Healing* (London, Ontario, 1990) provides an interesting parallel history of an eastern Canadian philanthropic society and its sanatorium in London, Ontario. Godfrey L. Gale, *The Changing Years* (Toronto, 1979) relates the story of the fight against tuberculosis at the Toronto Hospital (now known as West Park Hospital) in Weston, Ontario.

The historic medical situation in British Columbia receives attention from A.S. Monro, "The Medical History of British Columbia" (*Canadian Medical Association Journal* 1931-32); H.L. Burris,

Medical Saga: The Burris Clinic and Early Pioneers (Vancouver, 1967); and Glennis Zilm and Ethel Warbinek's "Early Tuberculosis Nursing in British Columbia" (*Canadian Journal of Nursing Research*, Fall 1995). For an understanding of tuberculosis nursing at the beginning of the century, see Ellen N. La Motte, *The Tuberculosis Nurse* (New York, 1985), originally published in 1915; for the mid-century, see Jessie G. Eyre, *Tuberculosis Nursing* (London, 1957). A patient's perspective is provided by Sybil MacFarlane's fine "Tranquille: Memories of the 1940s" in *British Columbia Historical News* (Winter 1991-92).

Primary sources are also extensive. The National Archives of Canada holds the records of the Military Hospitals Commission in RG 38. Records of the Canadian Association for the Prevention of Consumption and Other Forms of Tuberculosis and its successor, the Canadian Tuberculosis Association, are also at the NAC in MG 28 I 75. The British Columbia Lung Association holds the records of the Tranquille Tuberculosis Publicity Society and its successor, the British Columbia Tuberculosis Society. Also in the British Columbia Lung Association archives are informative memoirs by Esther Paulson and W.H. Hatfield, and what may be the only surviving complete collection of *The Tranquillian*.

Unfortunately, the records of the British Columbia Anti-Tuberculosis Society are divided among the British Columbia Lung Association, the Woodward Biomedical Library at the University of British Columbia, the British Columbia Archives and Record Service (BCARS), and the Kamloops Museum. Particularly useful for the early years of the society are the minute book and the Court of Governors book held by the Woodward Memorial Room at UBC, Additional MSS 1916 at BCARS, and the few letters at the Kamloops Archives. The annual reports published by the society are held by the British Columbia Lung Association, BCARS, and the Kamloops Museum.

BCARS holds the government records of the institution, most of them in the files of the provincial secretary. Particularly informative are GR 108 (Tranquille Sanatorium), GR 129 (Division of Tuberculosis Control), GR 496, GR 497, GR 2654, and GR 2866. The annual reports of the Tranquille Sanatorium are included in British Columbia

Sessional Papers for the years 1921 to 1935. After the reorganization of tuberculosis services, minimal information about the institution is found in the *Sessional Papers* in the annual reports of the Division of Tuberculosis Control from 1936 until 1959.

Newspapers provide details often not found elsewhere, but they should be used with caution. Information included here that pertains to the involvement of the community of Kamloops was often drawn from reports appearing in the *Kamloops Sentinel* (formerly the *Inland Sentinel*), the *Kamloops Standard*, the *Kamloops Telegram* and the *Kamloops Standard-Sentinel.* Other newspapers consulted were the *Victoria Colonist* and *Victoria Daily Times*, the *Vancouver News-Advertiser*, the *Vancouver Sun* and *Vancouver Province*, and, of course, *The Tranquillian.*

Finally, readers may be interested in the variety of comments on tuberculosis by artistic figures. See especially, John Keats, "Ode to a Nightingale" and "When I have fears that I might cease to be," and Thomas Mann's *The Magic Mountain.* Jimmy Rodgers "T.B. Blues" adds a musical dimension to the kind of poetry that circulated on the wards and in the "sanmags" of sanatoria throughout North America.

Index

A

B

C

D

E

F

G

H

I

J

K

L

M

N

O

P

Q

R

S

T

V

W